Jordaan,
Here's to a magical wor[ld]
crazy fuel filled
Bouncing [...]
[signature] x

C000153389

FUEL

Dean Jordaan,
Good Health & Happiness xxx
Enjoy!
[signature]

RƎTHINK PRESS

First published in Great Britain 2018
by Rethink Press (www.rethinkpress.com)

Cover image © Shutterstock / stockcreations
Interior design by Nelly Murariu

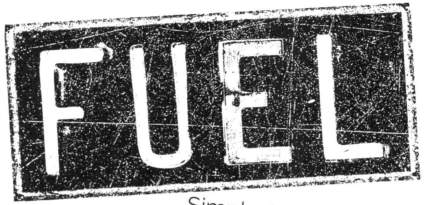

FUEL

Simple Juice and
Meal Plans to Help
You Get the **Bounce**
Back in Your Step

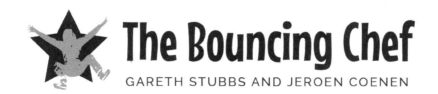

The Bouncing Chef

GARETH STUBBS AND JEROEN COENEN

BALANCE AND SIMPLICITY ARE KEY IN EVERYTHING. And so is Fun. Dance all night long and ALSO HAVE EARLY NIGHTS. *Practice yoga or stretch regularly* and have duvet days every now and then. Drink good wine with friends but **don't forget** your juices and water. Eat chocolate when your heart wants it and big salads when your body needs it. **LIVE HIGH** AND LOW, move and stay still, *sweat and relax*, laugh and cry, sing and be silent, READ BOOKS AND CHEESY MAGAZINES, watch TV and find a hobby. Pay it forward regularly. Wear underwear that makes you feel sexy. **Be kind to everyone you meet but don't tolerate rudeness —** instead, greet it with A SMILE because you've been there before.

MANIFESTO

Don't let anyone put you down and always find a way to compliment others, **EVEN IF IT MEANS SAYING NOTHING AT ALL.** *Embrace all sides of who you are.* **BE BRAVE, bold, SPONTANEOUS AND OUTRAGEOUS** and let that complement your ability to find silence, patience, humility, and peace. Embrace your emotions **BUT DON'T LET THEM CONTROL YOU.** **Do your best.** **HUG AND BE HUGGED.** Aim for balance and simplicity and don't get bogged down by the hype and drama. **Be firm and be free. BE MINDFUL AND MINDLESS.** *Make your own rules,* follow your own path, **live by your own decisions and choices,** and take responsibility for all that you do. **Take control and let go.** Don't let anybody else tell you how to live your life. **And above all else,** HAVE FUN AND **FEEL** GOOD AGAIN.

CONTENTS

This book is dedicated to each and every person who has sat down to have a meal in The Naya, out here at our retreat in Spain, and asked, 'What's in this?' or, 'How did you make this?' or, 'When are you going to write a recipe book?'

Introduction

Thanks for taking the time to pick up FUEL. We're really excited that this book has finally made its way into the world because writing it was one heck of a journey — one that we never imagined we'd take.

This might seem like just a recipe book, but it was created out of a passion to help people, to make a difference, and to show that it's possible to rebuild your life.

If you're looking for something to help you feel better about yourself, show you how to put better fuel into your body, give you tips and recipes to get you shifting weight, and leave you with a bounce in your step, happier and healthier, then guess what?

You're in the right place. In your hands, you've got the stuff to fuel your new life.

This book will not only challenge the way you approach eating, but also how you approach life as a whole. It will get you to question what you've been doing up until this point. And, more importantly, it will change the way you look at recipe books forever and help you put the bounce back into your step.

Who we are

We're Gareth and Jeroen, two regular guys from different backgrounds who had a shared dream: to one day have a retreat that would help people live healthy, balanced, and fulfilled lives. Together, we've faced some pretty tough challenges, but FUEL drives us to keep going. To keep pushing. To keep sharing. Most of all, it drives us to keep doing our best to help others rebuild their lives too.

As we became friends, we realised that the 'stuff' we'd been through in the past was something we 1) wanted to deal with and 2) wanted to help other people deal with too.

In 2014, when we decided to start D-Toxd, our health retreat in Spain, we never dreamt that it would lead to our putting this book together. Over the years, D-Toxd has become so much more than a health retreat thanks to our simple philosophy — *FUEL* — and the way of the Bouncing Chef.

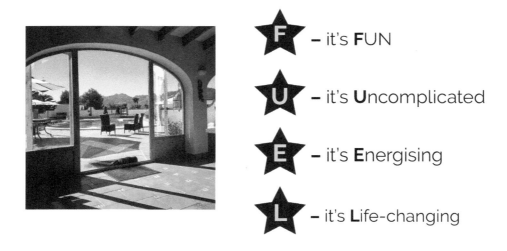

F – it's **F**UN

U – it's **U**ncomplicated

E – it's **E**nergising

L – it's **L**ife-changing

But you could say we became chefs by accident: the day we officially opened our retreat, the chef we'd hired to join our team never turned up — and people were paying to have healthy meals prepared for them. Since we didn't have time to look for a replacement, we dived in head first (as we typically do) and did the cooking ourselves.

What we do: the D-Toxd philosophy

If there's one thing that we're passionate about here at D-Toxd, it's embracing life. Take care of your body. Nurture your mind. Love your life. #daretobehealthy

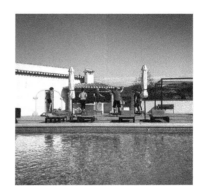

D-Toxd is a unique approach. It's designed to provide you with the opportunity (both online and in the physical world) to escape your busy life for a while so that you can truly recharge your batteries, get rid of excess weight, kick-start a new way of living, improve your health and fitness, reduce your stress levels, relax and have fun, ask questions and share insights, and, above all else, experience how simple and fun healthy living can really be.

We help you take care of your body by showing you what it needs (good, healthy, back-to-basics food, as well as exercise and rest and relaxation). We help you nurture your mind by sharing thought-provoking ideas and tools that encourage you to think differently. And we help you fall in love with your life in ways you never expected.

D-Toxd is about breaking free from the excuses and labels that restrict us, hold us back, and keep us stuck in that vicious cycle of dieting, weight loss, stress, and self-sabotage. It's about creating your own version of healthy, balanced living. It's not about extremes and radical lifestyle changes.

This version might offend and upset people. It might go against the grain, or even against reams and reams of research doing the rounds. It might test the myths and break through the barriers to show people how simple and fun being healthy can really be.

For us, being healthy isn't just about what we eat and what exercise we do. Through our free online communities, paid support groups, future online trainings, books and literature and retreat in Spain, our aim is to introduce people to a new way of life.

We know that life is for living and that if we want results, we need to take responsibility, create strategies, and go for them. Basically, we're regular people who do regular things and live balanced, healthy, happy and fulfilled lives — the D-Toxd way. Or, the FUEL way.

Why we do it

Both of us know what it's like to live an unhealthy lifestyle. Years of drug and alcohol abuse, neglecting our health and well-being, and generally living stress-filled lives led us individually to the point where we knew something had to change. We also know what it's like to reach rock bottom and be shaken awake to realise how truly special life is.

Change isn't easy, so we've spent the last fifteen years finding ways to make the complicated simple again, breaking down healthy living. We're not vegans, vegetarians, raw foodies or juice fanatics. Neither are we exercise junkies or yogis who meditate all day. We enjoy chocolate and wine, meat and potatoes, snacks and sneaky treats and lazy duvet days on the couch. We know that life is for living, and also that if we want results, we need to take responsibility, create strategies, and go for them.

Above all else, we believe that life is not about extremes and radical lifestyle changes. We choose to follow our own version of healthy, balanced living. Like we have said before, it's one that might offend and upset people. One that goes against the grain, or even against reams and reams of research doing the rounds. One that tests the myths and breaks through the barriers. One that shows people how simple and fun healthy, balanced living can really be — when we give ourselves permission to live this way.

A healthy lifestyle involves so much more than just eating the right foods; we must take care of our minds as well as our bodies. We've learned that physical health and mental health go hand in hand, and that balance is *vital*. Seeing the results that thousands of people have achieved as a result of making simple lifestyle changes has been pretty cool.

All of our meals are the result of research and experiments, tests and trials, and continually pushing ourselves to learn more. We're not chefs, and we've taught ourselves everything we do in the kitchen, so we guarantee this book contains no fancy jargon, technical terms, or meals that require a team of forty-eight in the kitchen. We prepare high-end, simple, healthy food in the shortest time possible because people lead busy lives and still need good, home-cooked food.

Over time, FUEL has become a way of life for the hundreds of people who have visited us. And for us, the cooking has become something we look forward to. For us, there is no greater pleasure in life than sharing a meal with people we care about. Eating is an experience to be treasured and valued and respected.

What you have in your hands right now is a simple, practical guide to our way of living and being healthy. If you implement the strategies we outline, you'll

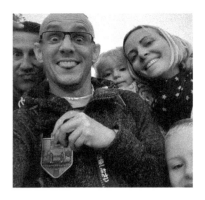

lose weight (if that's your goal). You'll have more energy. You'll enjoy eating more and have fun with food again. You'll enjoy more quality time with loved ones and friends. You'll approach life with a new outlook.

Above all else, you'll feel better and you'll find your own FUEL.

All About FUEL

It's not what you're eating — it's how you're eating it …

Before we get into anything food related, we'd like to share some foundational FUEL principles. Whatever your reasons for buying this book, we know that these principles will have a huge impact on your life.

Where does FUEL begin?

This isn't the time to dive deep into the reasons we developed the FUEL principles. But it all began when we embraced a few simple ideas. Ideas that, in fact, seemed too simple. We've spent the last four years refining these ideas so that you don't have to spend the next four years doing the same.

Many people embark on fitness plans that promise a beach body, unlimited energy, and renewed thinking. But it's easy to 'fail' diets and eating plans and workout regimes because they're too strict and too far removed from normal life. They ask us to deny ourselves the pleasures of life and make everything else a priority.

Some people think food is their problem. Some think it's lack of exercise. And for some people, it is as simple as that. Unfortunately, for most, this is *not* the truth.

For us, healthy living can be summed up in a simple scenario we've put together. Simplicity is what gives people the results they've been seeking for so long. Healthy living doesn't have to be complicated and it doesn't have to be hard work all the time. With just a few basic shifts in the way you approach food, and all that's involved with food, things start to change pretty quickly.

Imagine you had a newborn child to take care of and only forty-eight hours to teach him or her everything they needed to know to survive as a healthy grown-up in today's world.

Would you teach them to do all the things you're doing right now?

Would you teach them to speak to themselves the way you speak to yourself?

Would you push them as hard (or as little) as you push yourself?

What would you encourage them to do?

Understand this simple concept and it all falls into place.

You're in the *right place* and you're on the *right track* and starting today, things *can* be different.

Are you ready? Let's get our bounce on!

The FUEL Philosophy

At FUEL, we believe that happiness starts with how we FUEL our lives.

We put the fun back into healthy eating (and living) because at the end of the day, it's not what we eat but how we eat that matters most.

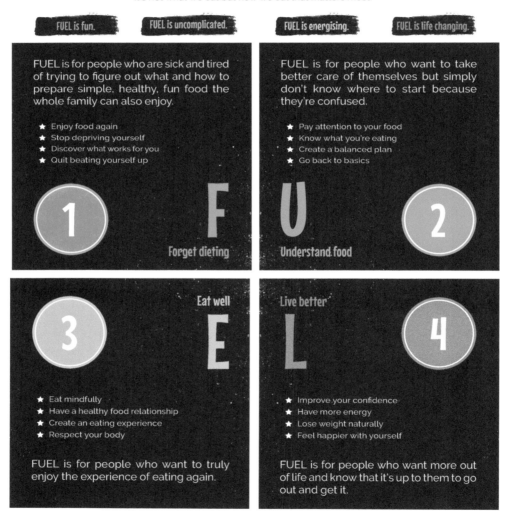

FUEL is fun.   **FUEL is uncomplicated.**

FUEL is for people who are sick and tired of trying to figure out what and how to prepare simple, healthy, fun food the whole family can also enjoy.

- ★ Enjoy food again
- ★ Stop depriving yourself
- ★ Discover what works for you
- ★ Quit beating yourself up

1

F Forget dieting

FUEL is energising.   **FUEL is life changing.**

FUEL is for people who want to take better care of themselves but simply don't know where to start because they're confused.

- ★ Pay attention to your food
- ★ Know what you're eating
- ★ Create a balanced plan
- ★ Go back to basics

2

U Understand food

Eat well

3

E

- ★ Eat mindfully
- ★ Have a healthy food relationship
- ★ Create an eating experience
- ★ Respect your body

FUEL is for people who want to truly enjoy the experience of eating again.

Live better

L

4

- ★ Improve your confidence
- ★ Have more energy
- ★ Lose weight naturally
- ★ Feel happier with yourself

FUEL is for people who want more out of life and know that it's up to them to go out and get it.

THE FOUR FUEL COMMANDMENTS

FUEL is about approaching things with a renewed way of thinking. Everything we do is about balance and simplicity. Embrace these few simple commandments and you'll put the bounce back into your step.

: Forget dieting

Enjoy food again

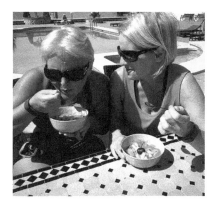

For many people, eating is a chore. It's easy to get caught up in a routine and then eat the same things over and over again. But eating can be exciting (and we'll provide recipes and plans to help you see this).

Always plate your food as if you are serving it to someone you love. Eating starts with the eyes, and if the food looks appealing, the body will be more ready to receive it. We salivate (the first part of the digestive process) before we even take the first mouthful.

Stop depriving yourself. Life is about enjoyment and fun. It's about doing things that bring us pleasure and make us feel good. Yet too often when it comes to food, we put way too much pressure on ourselves to get it right, to eat the 'right' things and not 'fall off the wagon', and deprive ourselves of things we enjoy.

If you're feeling overwhelmed by all the advice, one of the best things to do is free up your time. And the best way to do this is to plan ahead. Get a pen and paper and write down everything you think you need to do. Next, allocate times for these tasks and when doing so, work in some time for yourself, as well as time to exercise — fifteen to twenty minutes a day is sufficient. The main reason people don't get to the gym or do any exercise is because they don't schedule it in. They don't put themselves first.

If you don't take responsibility and control what you do in the time you have, everything will control you, time will run away, and you'll end up being way too hard on yourself.

Everything is good for you, in *moderation* — that's the key word.

Discover what works for you. Have you ever wondered why a hospital doesn't host parties? Or why a supermarket doesn't teach people physics and maths?

It's obvious: hospitals and supermarkets have specific purposes. They are unique and individual — just like each one of us. They know what works for them.

Even though the basic principles of healthy living might be the same for everyone, what works for one person might not work for another. Many studies say that 95% of people who go on diets regain all their weight and more within two years. Instead of going on a diet, find a balance that works for you. Enjoy the things you love in moderation. If you want to eat a bar of chocolate every day, do it, but take responsibility and understand that your body only does what it can do; you're responsible for the rest. You don't just shove any old fuel in your car, do you? So why do that with your body?

Find a definition of healthy living that you enjoy. Find one that gives you the results you're looking for. And in the process of creating and finding this, try different things because you never know what will work. When it does, have fun with it.

Not everyone likes celery, but that doesn't mean there's anything wrong with celery, right?

Quit beating yourself up

Guilt is a useless emotion that keeps us trapped in a cycle of never-ending frustration. Most of us are *way* too hard on ourselves, and often beat ourselves up over the simplest things.

On a physical level, guilt isn't good for us either. It produces all sorts of chemicals (and emotions) that have a negative effect on the body and, as a result, on what's going on physically when you're eating. This in turn affects how your body processes the fuel that you feed it.

It's harder to shift excess weight and rest properly when you're beating yourself up. And, quite simply, it stops you from having fun.

Remember this: where you are in your life right now, this point where you've decided to make changes – you didn't get here overnight. It might have taken you years to get here, so please, whatever you do, don't beat yourself up if you find that it takes time to start doing things differently.

⭐U: Understand food

Pay attention to your food

Eating is one of the most important things we do — food is the fuel that gets us through the day. But so often, we hear people say, 'Healthy food isn't that much fun', or 'Preparing my meals is boring'. When they approach a new way of eating, these thoughts are rolling round and round in their heads. As a result, instead of making changes, they quickly revert to old eating habits.

Take time reading through new recipes. Experiment with new ingredients. Try something different. Most importantly, simply pay a little extra attention to what you're eating, and you'll start to notice how it makes you feel.

Know what you're eating

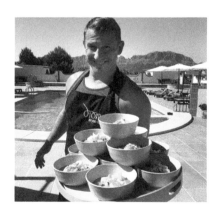

When you take time to prepare good, healthy meals, you know exactly what will be going into your body. You can see and smell how fresh your ingredients are.

Processed foods are full of things to keep them lasting longer. Most of us don't have any idea what these ingredients are, or where they came from. They may look healthy and the packaging might be appealing, but processed foods are stripped of nutrition and high in sugar. Instead of fuelling your body with something that's already been prepared for you, create your meals from scratch.

You'll see better results when you know exactly what you're eating, because you'll want to make better choices. Learn about basic nutrition and then find what works for you. And remember, there's nothing worse than a plate of brown slop; bright colours are inviting, and make you want to eat the food. Brightly coloured foods also contain more nutrients that are vital for good health. We need ALL food groups to live healthy, balanced lives.

Create a balanced plan

Life is about balance. We all have good days and bad days, ups and downs and everything in between. That's the joy of being human.

When it comes to balanced eating, we follow the 70/30 principle. We eat healthy meals 70% of the time — meals that contain loads of fresh fruits and vegetables. The rest of the time, we eat what we want, where we want, how we want.

And you know what? The more we follow this principle, and watch others do the same, the more positive changes we see.

'I don't have time to eat healthy', so many people say. Or, 'It takes too much effort'. Our simple response to these statements is 'Plan ahead'. Again, it's about taking responsibility. Shop online instead of going into the store, and spend the time you save travelling planning your meals — this way, you buy only what you need (you'll save money!), and you can relax knowing your meals for the week are in order.

Being prepared, you'll easily create balance and well-being in your life.

Go back to basics

Sometimes, becoming healthier is as simple (simple, not easy) as unlearning old habits and creating new ones.

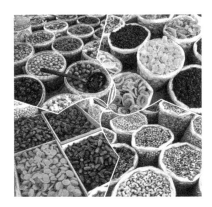

As humans, we often complicate things unnecessarily. We read stuff online and get overwhelmed. We see conflicting information and get confused.

Good, fresh food, regular exercise, plenty of water, and great company are the key ingredients for a happy and healthy life.

Try them.

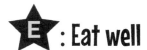 : Eat well

Eat mindfully

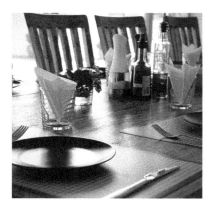

Eating time is for eating, nothing else. Don't work or scroll through social media sites while you eat. Sit and eat. Eat with your loved ones and enjoy the quality time.

Chew your food thoroughly — there's a reason why we have teeth in our mouth and not in our stomach. Your stomach is the 'holding tank' for the food, before it goes through the body, and chewing your food well helps your body digest it. Most of the digestive process takes place in the intestines.

Take a bite and then put your knife and fork down. Give yourself time to really taste the food you're eating. Swallow what you have just put into your mouth, and then pick up your knife and fork for the next mouthful.

Eating slowly is a simple way to avoid overeating. It takes twenty minutes for the brain to register that food has entered the system, so more often than not, we actually need a lot less than we really eat. Eat quickly, you eat more. Eat slowly, you eat less.

Your digestive system does more than digest food — it also absorbs emotions created as a result of watching TV and doing other distracting things. Create good emotions while eating and maximise the digestive process.

Have a healthy relationship with food

Take a look at your physical environment right now. Is it neat and tidy? Or chaotic and disorganised? Our environment (that place where we physically spend most of our time in, from home to socialising to work, and everywhere in between) plays a large part in our health as well. Always tidy the kitchen before you sit down to eat. You'll naturally have less energy afterwards, because the body uses it for digestion. Give yourself time to relax after the meal.

Are you surrounded by people who look after themselves? Who enjoying trying new recipes? Who like to live balanced lives? The people in our lives also contribute to the relationship that we have with food, and eating.

Create an eating experience

Create a ritual. Set the table and sit down and enjoy your food instead of mindlessly eating in front of the TV, or standing up in the kitchen. Not only will you eat less, you'll also start to understand when your body has had enough.

Always say grace. In other words, be thankful for what you are about to eat. Saying grace puts you in a positive frame of mind. Your frame of mind creates emotions within your body, which are (in effect) chemicals. The body absorbs these chemicals. Again, when you eat, not only are you digesting your food, you're also absorbing emotions.

What mood did you wake up in this morning? Cast your mind back to last night, when you had your last meal. What were you doing? How were you feeling? Nine times out of ten, your mood when you wake up in the morning can be linked directly to how you were feeling (or what you were saying and doing) when you sat down to eat your evening meal. Makes you think, doesn't it?

Respect your body

You get only one body this time around, so use it wisely. Treat it with respect. Take care of it.

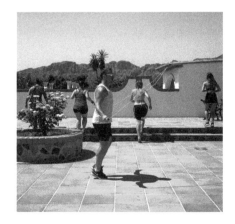

Move daily. Plain and simple, get out of breath every single day — but not so out of breath that you send your body into a state of shock. Get your heart rate up, but make sure you could still hold a conversation. A car uses fuel to move around; so does your body. Give it good fuel, use it wisely, and your body will reward you.

Get into the habit of eating at certain times. We put fuel in our cars when the gauge is low, but we don't always do the same with our bodies. When we don't eat regularly, the body starts to demand food and gets into the habit of having food 'on tap'. Creating regular eating times will help curb your hunger (and cravings) and get you more in touch with what you're putting into your body.

As you learn to respect your body, you will most definitely start to take better care of it.

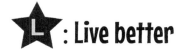 : Live better

Improve your confidence

Confidence is simply being comfortable in your own skin. It comes from deep down inside you. It's the ability to look at the person staring at you in the mirror and say, 'Hey, you and I, we got this, we can do this!'

It puts a bounce in your step and a smile on your face. It changes your posture and, in doing so, the way you feel.

Have more energy

If your body is full of good-quality foods, it will have more energy to do the things it's meant to do. If you're not eating quite right, the body will use excess energy to break down 'stuff' — something it shouldn't be doing.

When we eat well, energy is available for us to use.

Lose weight naturally

Weight loss is a natural by-product of healthy, balanced living.

Your body has one simple purpose: to keep you alive and healthy. It does whatever it can with whatever you give it to stick to that promise. If you don't pay attention to what you're feeding it, it will become harder and harder for the body to keep doing what it wants to do.

Change what you're giving it and the body will function the way it's meant to.

Feel happier with yourself

Think about what children are like when you pay attention to them and give them praise. They smile from ear to ear, they stand up straighter, and they do their best to do more of that thing that brought them praise.

The same goes for us. When we start taking care of ourselves, a ripple effect happens, from the inside out. This ripple has an effect on everything in our lives, including those around us.

Once you start to apply the principles we've discussed, you'll notice things shifting and changing. We can't wait for you to experience this.

GET PREPARED: THE MEAL PLANS

The hardest part of cooking is getting yourself ready. We can help you with that. We keep our recipes short, sweet, and to the point, so you'll be able to do what we do in our kitchen.

We've put together a few plans that you can follow at home. In our experience, most people have great intentions but give up before they even begin because they simply don't take time to sit down and make a plan. In fact, most people probably spend more time planning parties or holidays than they do their meals, and then they wonder why they are where they are in terms of their health.

Some of the meal plans involve what we do at the retreat every week – they follow exactly the same format that we use when people spend time with us (three days of juicing followed by four days of healthy, home-cooked meals). Some are designed for those wishing to try something different, and some are for those who want to make meals the whole family can enjoy.

Whichever plan you choose, we recommend starting it on a Sunday — this way, you'll have enough time to get prepared in advance.

Here's a breakdown of the plans:

The seven-day fruit and veg juice plan

For seven days, drink juices and smoothies that combine a variety of fruits and vegetables. If you're new to juicing, don't worry — these recipes aren't too hardcore.

The seven-day alkaline juice plan

This plan is similar to the first one, but involves less sweet stuff. It's ideal for people wishing to live a more alkaline lifestyle. If you haven't juiced before, we recommend trying some of these out before committing to the plan, as they can be quite strong.

The five-day juice and soup detox plan

For people who want to give their digestive systems a break but aren't quite ready to do a full seven-day juice cleanse, this plan includes smoothie bowls and soup as well. We have also included some suggestions for easy snack juices where you would simply use one of the ingredients listed. You won't feel like you're missing out on anything.

The four-week plan

This is a twenty-eight-day programme with a wide variety of meals to choose from and a simple list of ingredients. It's been put together to give your body everything it needs while keeping it on its toes with variety — something that's easy to forget about.

Week One – seven-day juice and meal plan: Week One is an example of the exact programme we follow at the retreat. You'll start with a three-day juice cleanse to give your digestive system a break, and move on to delicious, simple, and healthy meals and snacks.

Week Two – seven-day meal plan: Week Two offers meals and snacks the whole family can enjoy.

Week Three – seven-day juice and meal plan: Week Three is another plan that follows the retreat's structure.

Week Four – seven-day meal plan: Week Four is also about meals and snacks the whole family can enjoy.

The seven-day clean-eating plan

This plan is ideal for people recovering from illness or stress. The meals and snacks are alkaline-based, which means they're lighter, and slightly easier to digest.

Your next step is simple, really.

Choose one and get started!

The seven-day fruit and veg juice plan

DAY	BREAKFAST	LUNCH	DINNER
Day 1: Sunday	Morning Bliss	P-Arrot	Ginger Bam Plus
Day 2: Monday	Red Robot	D-Toxd Alkalise	Berry Kiss
Day 3: Tuesday	Amber Agent	Popeye's Detox	D-Toxd Tonic
Day 4: Wednesday	'Pear' Fect	Lemon Zing	D-Toxd Detox Boost
Day 5: Thursday	Vampire's Dream	Fruit Salad	Immune Booster
Day 6: Friday	Green Giant	Pineapple Blast	'Bloody' Mary
Day 7: Saturday	Breakfast Smoothie	Digest Ade	Red Mud

The seven-day alkaline juice plan

DAY	BREAKFAST	LUNCH	DINNER
Day 1: Sunday	Sweet Tooth	D- Toxd Rainbow	Power Up
Day 2: Monday	Fresh Start	Meta Boost	Green Goblin
Day 3: Tuesday	Greenie Meanie	Field of Dreams	Mega Mix
Day 4: Wednesday	Purple Rain	Lemon Zing	D-Toxd Leprechaun
Day 5: Thursday	Kick Starter	D-Toxd Alkalise	Beet Ade
Day 6: Friday	Get It Moving	Red Raindrop	Salad
Day 7: Saturday	Pharmacia	Forest	'Bloody' Mary

The five-day juice and soup detox plan

DAY	BREAKFAST	SNACK	LUNCH	SNACK	DINNER
Day 1	Juices Morning Bliss	Snack juice Apple, ginger, lemon, and coconut water	Juices P-arrot	Snack juice Cucumber, lime, orange, and mint	Juices Ginger Bam Plus
Day 2	Juices 'Pear' Fect	Snack juice Cucumber, lime, orange, and mint	Juices D-Toxd Tonic	Snack juice Apple, ginger, lemon, and coconut water	Juices Immune Booster
Day 3	Juices Popeye's Detox	Snack juice Apple, ginger, lemon, and coconut water	Juices Digest Ade	Snack juice Cucumber, lime, orange, and mint	Juices Ginger Bam Plus
Day 4	Smoothie bowls Bana Cado	Snack juice Cucumber, lime, orange, and mint	Juices P-Arrot	Snack juice Apple, ginger, lemon, and coconut water	Soups Detox superfood green vegetable soup
Day 5	Smoothie bowls Banana Berry	Snack juice Apple, ginger, lemon, and coconut water	Juices Popeye's Detox	Snack juice Cucumber, lime, orange, and mint	Soups Courgette, pea, and mint soup

The four-week plan

Week One – seven-day juice and meal plan

DAY	BREAKFAST	SNACK	LUNCH	SNACK	DINNER
Day 1: Sunday Juice Day	**Juices** Morning Bliss	**Snack juice** Glass of 100% natural juice of choice	**Juices** P-Arrot	**Soups** Cup of D-Toxd vegetable soup (blended)	**Juices** Ginger Bam Plus
Day 2: Monday Juice Day	**Juices** Red Robot	**Snack juice** Glass of 100% natural juice of choice	**Juices** D-Toxd Alkalise	**Soups** Cup of D-Toxd vegetable soup (blended)	**Juices** Berry Kiss
Day 3: Tuesday Juice Day	**Juices** Amber Agent	**Snack juice** Glass of 100% natural juice of choice	**Juices** Popeye's Detox	**Soups** Cup of D-Toxd vegetable soup (blended)	**Juices** D-Toxd Tonic
Day 4: Wednesday Meals	**Smoothie bowls** Bana Cado	**Snacks, treats, and desserts** Energy ball and piece of fruit	**Soups** D-Toxd vegetable soup	**Snacks, treats, and desserts** Birdseed bar	**Meals** D-Toxd mushroom Alfredo with courgette spaghetti
Day 5: Thursday Meals	**Smoothie bowls** Green Garden	**Snacks, treats, and desserts** Birdseed bar	**Soups** Chilli butternut squash and ginger soup	**Snacks, treats, and desserts** Energy ball and piece of fruit	**Meals** Lentil cottage pie with mustard sweet potato mash
Day 6: Friday Meals	**Smoothie bowls** Banana Split	**Snacks, treats, and desserts** Energy ball and piece of fruit	**Soups** Leek, asparagus, and baby potato soup	**Snacks, treats, and desserts** Birdseed bar	**Meals** Sweet potato and chickpea curry
Day 7: Saturday Meals	**Breakfasts** Spanish pepper, spinach, and feta tortilla	**Snacks, treats, and desserts** Birdseed bar	**Salads** Avocado, asparagus, and broccoli salad	**Snacks, treats, and desserts** Energy ball and piece of fruit	**Meals** Thai baked fish parcels **Snacks, treats, and desserts** Avocado and pistachio ice cream

Week Two – seven-day meal plan

DAY	BREAKFAST	SNACK	LUNCH	SNACK	DINNER
Day 1 **Sunday**	**Smoothie bowls** Caribbean Bowl	**Snacks, treats, and desserts** Courgette and apple muffins	**Soups** Carrot and red pepper soup	**Snacks, treats, and desserts** Apricot energy bar	**Meals** Broccoli and chickpea burgers with courgette spaghetti and tomato sauce
Day 2 **Monday**	**Breakfasts** Overnight oats	**Snacks, treats, and desserts** Apricot energy bar	**Salads** Apple and carrot spinach slaw	**Snacks, treats, and desserts** Courgette and apple muffins	**Meals** D-Toxd chilli sin carne
Day 3 **Tuesday**	**Breakfasts** Breakfast parfait	**Snacks, treats, and desserts** Courgette and apple muffins	**Soups** Roast tomato and basil soup	**Snacks, treats, and desserts** Apricot energy bar	**Meals** Broccoli and cashew nut pesto sauce with mushrooms
Day 4 **Wednesday**	**Breakfasts** Breakfast egg muffins	**Snacks, treats, and desserts** Apricot energy bar	**Salads** Mandi's warm mackerel and cannellini bean salad	**Snacks, treats, and desserts** Courgette and apple muffins	**Meals** Stuffed red peppers
Day 5 **Thursday**	**Breakfasts** Quinoa chia porridge	**Snacks, treats, and desserts** Courgette and apple muffins	**Soups** Courgette, pea, and cannellini bean soup	**Snacks, treats, and desserts** Apricot energy bar	**Meals** Thai sweet potato curry
Day 6 **Friday**	**Breakfasts** Chocolate yogurt sundae	**Snacks, treats, and desserts** Apricot energy bar	**Meals** Tuna and apple wraps	**Snacks, treats, and desserts** Courgette and apple muffins	**Meals** Miripiri's beef stroganoff and green beans
Day 7 **Saturday**	**Smoothie bowls** Spinach and Blueberry	**Snacks, treats, and desserts** Courgette and apple muffins	**Soups** Potato, asparagus, pea, and mint soup	**Snacks, treats, and desserts** Apricot energy bar	**Meals** Lemon, bacon, and cherry-tomato baked cod **Snacks, treats, and desserts** Courgette and almond brownies with caramel sauce

Week Three – seven-day juice and meal plan

DAY	BREAKFAST	SNACK	LUNCH	SNACK	DINNER
Day 1: Sunday Juice Day	**Juices** 'Pear' Fect	**Snack juice** Glass of 100% natural juice of choice	**Juices** Lemon Zing	**Soups** Cup of soup of choice (blended)	**Juices** D-Toxd detox boost
Day 2: Monday Juice Day	**Juices** Vampire's Dream	**Snack juice** Glass of 100% natural juice of choice	**Juices** Fruit Salad	**Soups** Cup of soup of choice (blended)	**Juices** 'Bloody' Mary
Day 3: Tuesday Juice Day	**Juices** Green Giant	**Snack juice** Glass of 100% natural juice of choice	**Juices** Pineapple Blast	**Soups** Cup of soup of choice (blended)	**Juices** Immune Booster
Day 4: Wednesday Meals	**Smoothie bowls** Vanilla Strawberry	**Snacks, treats, and desserts** Handful of D-Toxd mixed nuts	**Soups** Courgette, carrot, and sweet potato soup	**Snacks, treats, and desserts** Red pepper hummus and vegetable sticks	**Meals** Roast butternut squash and red pepper sauce
Day 5: Thursday Meals	**Smoothie bowls** Tropical Smoothie	**Snacks, treats, and desserts** Coconut delight	**Soups** Roast red pepper and tomato soup	**Snacks, treats, and desserts** Pesto hummus and vegetable sticks	**Meals** Banana and kidney bean wraps
Day 6: Friday Meals	**Smoothie bowls** Banana Berry	**Snacks, treats, and desserts** Handful of mixed nuts and piece of fruit	**Soups** Cauli-broc mustard soup	**Snacks, treats, and desserts** Coconut delight	**Meals** Anne's oven-baked aubergine with olive and caper sauce
Day 7: Saturday Meals	**Breakfasts** Scrambled tofu	**Snacks, treats, and desserts** Handful of mixed nuts and piece of fruit	**Salads** Chickpea, avocado, and feta salad	**Snacks, treats, and desserts** Coconut delight	**Meals** Tangy sweet and spicy chicken **Snacks, treats, and desserts** Banana ice cream

Week Four – seven-day meal plan

DAY	BREAKFAST	SNACK	LUNCH	SNACK	DINNER
Day 1: Sunday Juice Day	**Smoothie bowls** Peanut butter and chocolate	**Snacks, treats, and desserts** Cranberry granola bar	**Salads** Spinach, avocado, and pepper salad with grilled chicken	**Snacks, treats, and desserts** D-Toxd fruit salad and yogurt	**Meals** Vegetable lasagne
Day 2: Monday Juice Day	**Breakfasts** Smoked salmon on toast	**Snacks, treats, and desserts** Piece of fruit	**Soups** Chilli chickpea and lemon soup	**Snacks, treats, and desserts** Cranberry granola bar	**Meals** Baked salsa sweet potato bowls
Day 3: Tuesday Juice Day	**Breakfasts** Quinoa fruit bowl	**Snacks, treats, and desserts** Cranberry granola bar	**Salads** D-Toxd baked beans and salad wrap	**Snacks, treats, and desserts** Guacamole and rye bread	**Meals** Oven-baked sea bass with sweet potato chilli mash
Day 4; Wednesday Meals	**Breakfasts** Chocolate yogurt sundae	**Snacks, treats, and desserts** Guacamole and rye bread	**Soups** Carrot and coriander soup	**Snacks, treats, and desserts** Cranberry granola bar	**Meals** Thai red vegetable curry
Day 5: Thursday Meals	**Smoothie bowls** Courgette and Coconut	**Snacks, treats, and desserts** Cranberry granola bar	**Salads** Courgette with creamy avocado mustard dressing	**Snacks, treats, and desserts** Piece of fruit	**Meals** Pumpkin and pea risotto
Day 6: Friday Meals	**Breakfasts** Breakfast wrap	**Snacks, treats, and desserts** D-Toxd fruit salad and yogurt	**Soups** Spicy sweet potato soup	**Snacks, treats, and desserts** Cranberry granola bar	**Meals** Roast fennel and onion with mushroom, broccoli, and avocado cream
Day 7: Saturday Meals	**Smoothie bowls** Mango Delight	**Snacks, treats, and desserts** Cranberry granola bar	**Soups** Miripiri's warm chickpea and chorizo salad	**Snacks, treats, and desserts** Piece of fruit	**Meals** Grilled Parmesan chicken and Smoked Paprika & Garlic Tomato sauce **Snacks, treats, and desserts** Avocado and basil panna cotta

The seven-day clean-eating plan

DAY	BREAKFAST	SNACK	LUNCH	SNACK	DINNER
Day 1: Sunday Juice Day	**Smoothie bowls** Bana Cado	**Snacks, treats, and desserts** Apricot energy bar	**Soups** Courgette, carrot, and sweet potato soup	**Snacks, treats, and desserts** Red pepper hummus and vegetable sticks	**Meals** Roast butternut squash and red pepper sauce with courgette spaghetti
Day 2: Monday Juice Day	**Breakfasts** Breakfast tortilla	**Snacks, treats, and desserts** Mixed nuts and fruit	**Salads** D-Toxd baked beans and salad wrap	**Snacks, treats, and desserts** Apricot energy bar	**Meals** Baked aubergine with tomato and olive sauce
Day 3: Tuesday Juice Day	**Breakfasts** Seed cereal and yogurt	**Snacks, treats, and desserts** Apricot energy bar	**Soups** Cauli-broc mustard soup	**Snacks, treats, and desserts** Pesto hummus and vegetable sticks	**Meals** Tangy sweet and spicy chicken with carrot and courgette noodles
Day 4: Wednesday Meals	**Smoothie bowls** Banana Berry	**Snacks, treats, and desserts** Mixed nuts and fruit	**Salads** Spinach, avocado, and pepper salad	**Snacks, treats, and desserts** Apricot energy bar	**Meals** Thai vegetable curry
Day 5: Thursday Meals	**Breakfasts** Overnight oats	**Snacks, treats, and desserts** Apricot energy bar	**Salads** Tomato and chickpea Salad	**Snacks, treats, and desserts** Red pepper hummus and vegetable sticks	**Meals** Oven-baked sea bass with sweet potato chilli mash
Day 6: Friday Meals	**Breakfasts** Seed cereal and yogurt	**Snacks, treats, and desserts** Mixed nuts and fruit	**Soups** Courgette, carrot, and sweet potato soup	**Snacks, treats, and desserts** Apricot energy bar	**Meals** D-Toxd chilli sin carne
Day 7: Saturday Meals	**Smoothie bowls** Banana Split	**Snacks, treats, and desserts** Apricot energy bar	**Soups** Cauli-broc mustard soup	**Snacks, treats, and desserts** D-Toxd fruit salad and yogurt	**Meals** Broccoli and chickpea burgers with courgette spaghetti and tomato sauce

Stuff to get you going

At our retreat, we don't have an industrial kitchen with all the latest gadgets and appliances, and we don't have a huge pantry filled with exotic ingredients. In fact, quite the opposite. We run D-Toxd like a home. It's a place where people can feel comfortable and taken care of.

We have a selection of pots and pans, some basic kitchen utensils, and a small four-plate gas stove that has served us well. We also have blenders (both stationary and handheld), a juicer, and a food processor — and with all of these items, we have proved to ourselves that you don't need anything fancy to prepare and serve good, healthy food.

We've broken down the ingredients you'll need into two categories: store cupboard ingredients and bought ingredients.

Store cupboard ingredients

These are the ingredients that can be bought in advance, stored, and used in loads of different meals. These items are *not* included in the shopping lists (mentioned below). Please note that you don't need to have all of these, and they aren't all used in all of the recipes.

Almond or soy milk

Apple cider vinegar

Baking powder

Balsamic vinegar

Bay leaves

Black pepper (we use peppercorns in a grinder)

Breadcrumbs

Butter (unsalted)

Cacao powder

Cayenne pepper

Chia seeds

Coconut oil

Coriander seeds

Cumin seeds

Curry powder of your choice

Dried chilli flakes

Dried mixed herbs

Dried oats

Dried oregano

Dried tarragon

Dried thyme

English mustard

Flour – almond, chickpea, or rice

Ground cinnamon

Ground cumin

Ground ginger

Ground pimento

Ground turmeric

Honey

Nutmeg

Olive oil

Quinoa

Red wine vinegar

Salt – Himalayan rock salt or sea salt flakes are best

Sesame seeds

Smoked paprika

Soya sauce

Tahini

Tomato puree

Vanilla essence

Vegetable stock cubes

Wholegrain mustard

Bought ingredients

On our website, you'll find a 'bought ingredients' shopping list for each of the meal plans. After selecting your plan, download the bought ingredients list and get all your shopping done in one go. At the retreat, we plan all our meals ahead of time and buy these ingredients weekly.

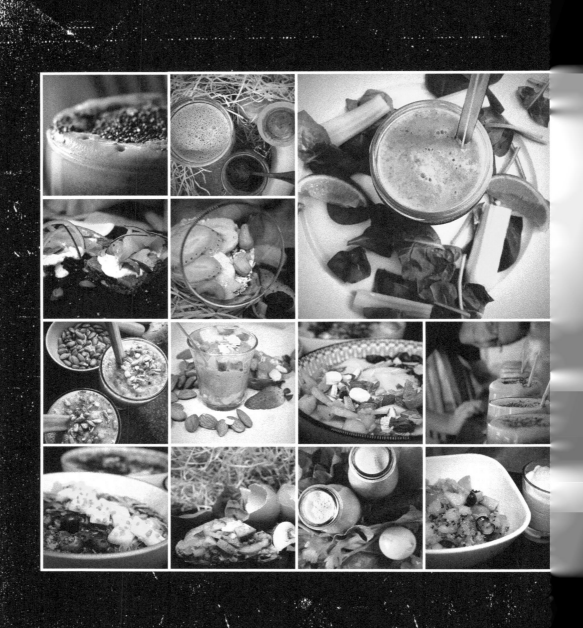

FUEL TO START YOUR DAY: JUICES, SMOOTHIE BOWLS, AND HEALTHY BREAKFASTS

Your first meal of the day sets up the nutritional highway you follow as the day unfolds. Your energy levels, cravings, and (to some extent) emotions can often be linked to this meal.

Eating well isn't just about green things and juices. This chapter includes a variety of breakfast options, so you can create a healthy first meal of the day that suits you.

Recipes in this section

JUICES		SMOOTHIE BOWLS	BREAKFASTS
A Bowl of Breakfast	Immune Booster	Bana Cado	Breakfast egg muffins
Amber Agent	Kick Starter	Banana Berry	Breakfast parfait
Beet Ade	Lemon Zing	Banana Split	Breakfast tortilla
Berry Kiss	Mega Mix	Caribbean Bowl	Breakfast wrap
'Bloody' Mary	Meta Boost	Courgette and Coconut	Chocolate yogurt sundae
Breakfast Smoothie	Morning Bliss	Green Garden	D-Toxd C:Real
Digest Ade	P-Arrot	Mango Delight	Overnight oats
D-Toxd Alkalise	'Pear' Fect	Peanut Butter and Chocolate	Quinoa chia porridge
D-Toxd Breakfast Booster	Pharmacia	Spinach and Blueberry	Quinoa fruit bowl
D-Toxd Detox Boost	Pina Colada	Tropical Smoothie	Scrambled tofu
D-Toxd Leprechaun	Pineapple Kick	Vanilla Strawberry	Seed cereal
D-Toxd Rainbow	Pine Blast		Smoked salmon on toast
D-Toxd Tonic	Popeye's Detox		Spanish pepper, spinach, and feta tortilla
Field of Dreams	Power Up		
Forest	Purple Rain		
Fresh Start	Red Mud		
Fruit Salad	Red Raindrop		
Get It Moving	Red Robot		
Ginger Bam Plus	Salad		
Green Giant	Sweet Tooth		
Green Goblin	Vampire's Dream		
Greenie Meanie			

Juicing: A brief introduction

Drinking juices and smoothies is a great way to flush your body with nutrients. You can pack them full of fresh, healthy ingredients, and if you've been through a period of illness or stress, they're a great way to give your digestive system a break. Quite simply, drinking juices and/or smoothies is the simplest and most fun way to get your daily nutrients.

Juices are prepared using a machine called a juicer, which extracts the juice of certain fruits and vegetables and sets aside the fibre and pulp.

Smoothies are prepared by placing either whole fruits and/or vegetables into a blender (or a specific smoothie-making machine such as a NutriBullet) or a combination of whole items and juiced ones. They contain the fruits' fibre and are therefore a lot thicker.

The trick with creating juices and smoothies is to get your blend of fruit and vegetables right — too much fruit and you'll flood your body with sugar; too much veg will be tough to handle taste-wise if you aren't used to it. That's not to say that you can't have a juice or smoothie that's mostly fruit every now and then. The danger lies in drinking that same beverage over and over and over again.

Sometimes, you're going to want more fruit than veg — it's natural. You're human. The important thing is to be aware of what you're putting into the juices and smoothies you create, and to find that balance of ingredients.

Watch out for our indicators. They'll let you know what to expect from each of our juices and smoothies.

 The sweet choice
New to juicing and want to make sure you enjoy your drink? This one is ideal for you — it's sweet and easy on the palate.

 The less-sweet choice
This one uses less fruit; it's tasty yet not too sweet.

 The hardcore choice
If you're looking for the most alkaline (and lowest-calorie) choice, go for this. But beware! It might take some getting used to.

We don't believe in extended periods of juicing (unless there are extreme circumstances). While it does contribute to weight loss, it's not sustainable in the long run. If you have tried other diets or food replacement programmes that haven't worked for you, it may be because your body "clings on' to everything that it gets once it receives solid food again, which defeats the purpose.

However, shocks to the system every now and then are a great way to kick-start the natural bodily functions and, as mentioned, give the digestive system a break. That's why we encourage people to do a juice and smoothie cleanse every now and then. We do three days of juicing at our retreat in Spain.

In this book, we're not going to debate whether juices are better than smoothies, or whether juicers are better than blenders. Each has its pros and cons. Our plans are about making personal choices and going with whichever options suit you best.

As stated in our manifesto, we don't get caught up in hype – and by hype, we mean all that 'quick fix, magical cure' jargon around. We believe that juicing is about not only giving your body what it needs, but also about enjoying what you put into your body.

If you haven't tried juicing, give it a go. After three days at the retreat, people who have never juiced before feel all its benefits, and they return home able to incorporate it into their lives in a balanced way. They don't juice every single day — and neither do we. But we do encourage you to have a juice or smoothie for breakfast at least three times a week, for a good dose of FUEL.

Things to remember

Hard fruits and vegetables, such as apples, lemons, pineapples, melons, beetroots, carrots, etc, go in the juicer.

Soft fruits, such as bananas, strawberries and other berries, mangos (pips removed), avocados (pips and skin removed), etc, go in the blender. Fresh baby spinach leaves can also be thrown in the blender.

★

When using ingredients with rinds, it's often better to peel them, as the rind contains oils that will give the drink a bitter taste – always peel oranges, limes, and grapefruits.

★

Wash your juicer or blender *straight away* after using — it will save you time. There's nothing worse than cleaning a sticky juicer or blender.

★

Place a compostable plastic bag in your waste container — you'll have one less thing to wash.

If making a drink for later on, immediately place it in the fridge, in an airtight container. When juices or smoothies are exposed to air and light, they lose their nutritional value.

If you want to freeze your drink, immediately place it in the freezer in a plastic bottle. Take it out an hour or two before drinking and wrap it in a tea towel so that it isn't exposed to too much light. Make sure you leave the lid off when you first put it in the freezer. Sealed bottles can expand and 'explode'.

If making a drink to take with you, immediately place it in a thermos or aluminium flask and seal it.

Juices

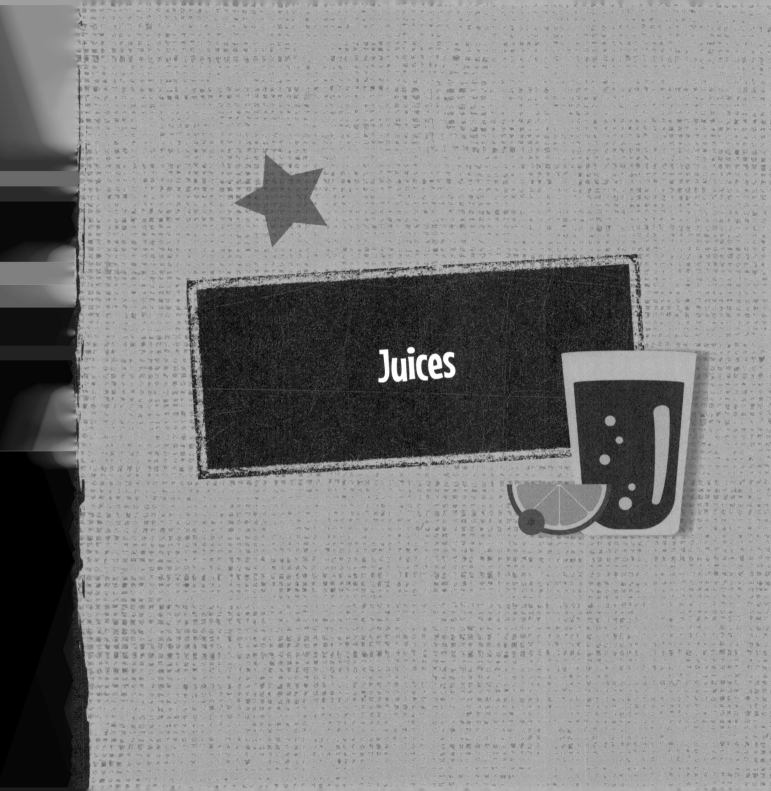

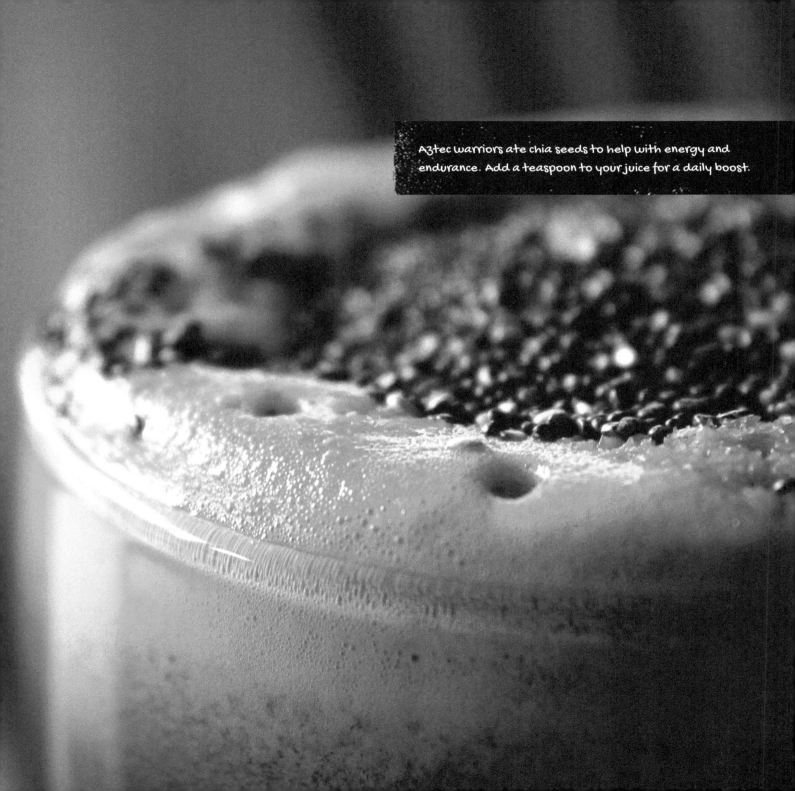

Aztec warriors ate chia seeds to help with energy and endurance. Add a teaspoon to your juice for a daily boost.

A Bowl Of Breakfast	Amber Agent	Beet Ade	Berry Kiss
2 apples	1 apple	2 beetroots	1 apple
1 banana	3 carrots	½ English cucumber	2 carrots
1 courgette	2 celery sticks	2 large carrots	1 courgette
1 handful of strawberries	1 courgette	1 small chunk of ginger	½ lemon
3 tablespoons of Greek yogurt	½ English cucumber	1 lemon	1 pear
1 tsp of bee pollen	1 small chunk of ginger	------------------	1 handful of strawberries
1 tsp of cacao powder	½ lemon	★ Juice all ingredients	½ avocado
------------------	½ avocado		------------------
★ Juice apples and courgette	------------------		★ Juice apple, carrots, courgette, lemon, and pear
★ Blend with remaining ingredients until smooth and creamy	★ Juice apple, carrots, celery, courgette, cucumber, ginger, and lemon		★ Blend with strawberries and avocado until smooth and creamy
	★ Blend with avocado until smooth and creamy		

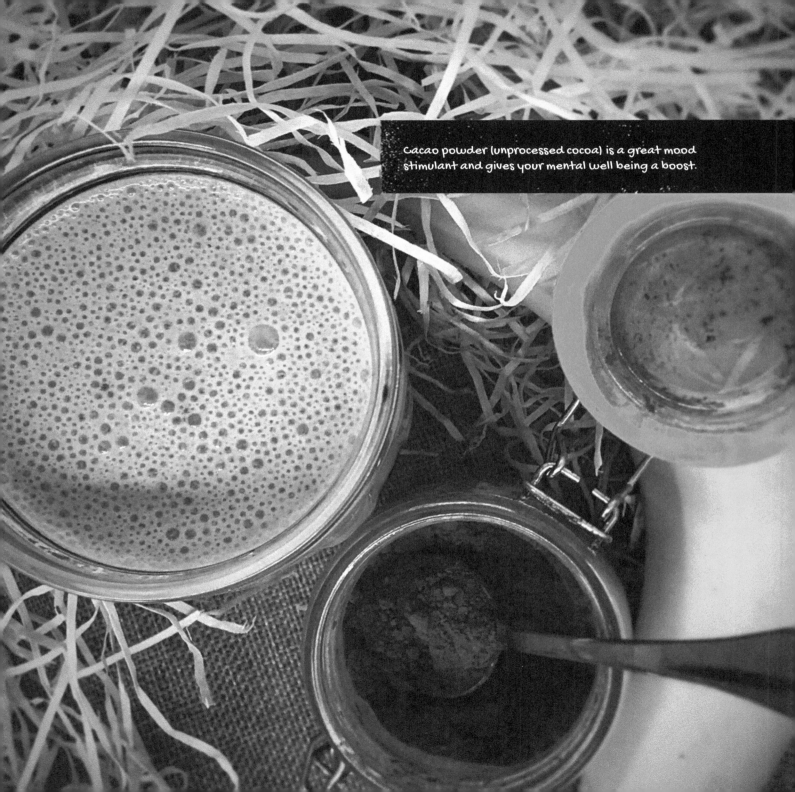

Cacao powder (unprocessed cocoa) is a great mood stimulant and gives your mental well being a boost.

'Bloody' Mary	Breakfast Smoothie	Digest Ade	D-Toxd Alkalise
½ beetroot	2 apples	2 apples	1 apple
2 carrots	1 banana	2 celery sticks	3 celery sticks
1 courgette	2 large carrots	½ English cucumber	1 courgette
2 tomatoes	1 courgette	½ fennel bulb	½ English cucumber
½ lemon	1 handful of strawberries	1 small chunk of ginger	1 small chunk of ginger
½ avocado	1 teaspoon of bee pollen	1 lime (peeled)	1 lime (peeled)
pinch of sea salt		1 orange (peeled)	3 handfuls of spinach
chilli (optional for heat)		1 handful of spinach	1 teaspoon spirulina (optional)

'Bloody' Mary

- ★ Juice beetroot, carrots, courgette, lemon and tomatoes
- ★ Blend with avocado, sea salt and chilli (if using) until smooth and creamy

Breakfast Smoothie

- ★ Juice apples, carrots, and courgette
- ★ Blend with strawberries, banana and bee pollen until smooth and creamy

Digest Ade

- ★ Juice all ingredients

D-Toxd Alkalise

- ★ Juice all ingredients
- ★ Blend with spirulina (if using), or stir in well

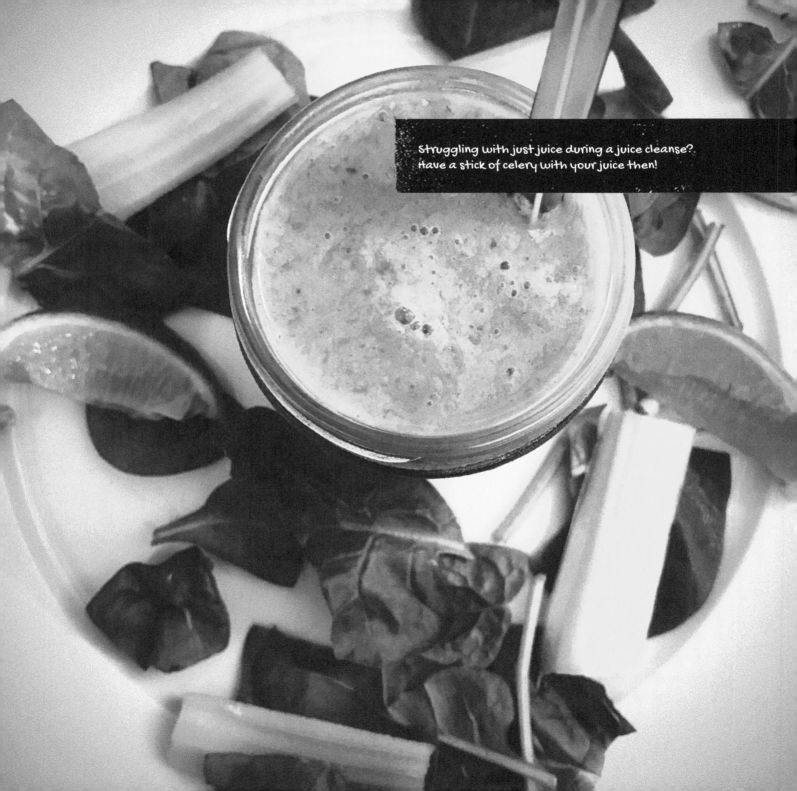

Struggling with just juice during a juice cleanse?
Have a stick of celery with your juice then!

D-Toxd Breakfast Booster	D-Toxd Detox Boost	D-Toxd Leprechaun	D-Toxd Rainbow
1 apple	1 apple	1 broccoli stem	2 carrots
1 courgette	1 broccoli stem	2 celery sticks	1 celery stick
1 banana	1 large carrot	½ English cucumber	½ English cucumber
½ cup of almond milk	2 celery sticks	1 medium chunk of ginger	1 small chunk of ginger
2 tablespoons Greek yogurt	½ courgette	1 lime (peeled)	½ lemon
1 small handful of oats	½ English cucumber	1 large handful of spinach	1 small handful of fresh parsley
1 handful of strawberries	1 small chunk of ginger	1 tomato	1 red pepper
	½ lemon	1 teaspoon of spirulina (optional)	-------------------
-------------------	1 small handful of fresh parsley	-------------------	★ Juice all ingredients
★ Juice apple and courgette	½ yellow pepper	★ Juice all ingredients	
★ Blend with remaining ingredients until smooth and creamy	½ avocado	★ Blend with spirulina (if using), or stir in well	

	★ Juice all ingredients except the avocado		
	★ Blend with avocado until smooth and creamy		

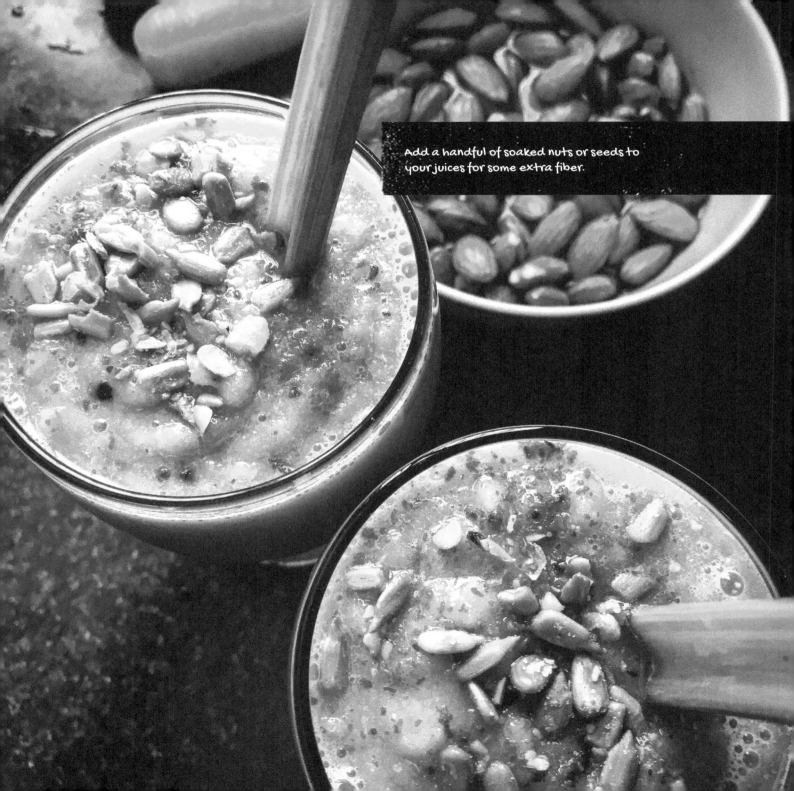

Add a handful of soaked nuts or seeds to your juices for some extra fiber.

D-Toxd Tonic	Field Of Dreams	Forest	Fresh Start
1 apple	150g white cabbage	1 apple	2 beetroots
1 beetroot	1 courgette	½ English cucumber	3 large carrots
1 broccoli stem	½ English cucumber	2 celery sticks	½ English cucumber
1 large carrot	1 small chunk of ginger	1 small chunk of ginger	1 small chunk of ginger
2 celery sticks	1 lemon	1 large handful of kale	1 lemon
½ English cucumber	1 small handful of fresh parsley	1 large handful of lettuce	1 red pepper
1 small chunk of ginger	3 large handfuls of spinach	1 lime (peeled)	½ avocado (optional)
½ lemon	- - - - - - - - - - - - - - - - - - -	1 small handful of fresh parsley	- - - - - - - - - - - - - - - - - - -
1 small handful of fresh parsley	★ Juice all ingredients	1 large handful of spinach	★ Juice all ingredients except the avocado
- - - - - - - - - - - - - - - - - - -		- - - - - - - - - - - - - - - - - - -	★ Blend with avocado until smooth and creamy
★ Juice all ingredients		★ Juice all ingredients	

If you don't like the froth (or head) on your juice, simply scoop it off!

Fruit Salad	Get It Moving	Ginger Bam Plus	Green Giant
1 apple	150g white cabbage	2 apples	1 apple
1 tsp of bee pollen	½ English cucumber	½ beetroot	1 broccoli stem
½ English cucumber	1 tsp of flax seed	2 carrots	2 celery sticks
1 small chunk of ginger	1 small chunk of ginger	½ courgette	½ English cucumber
1 lime (peeled)	½ lemon	1 large chunk of ginger	1 small chunk of ginger
1 large orange (peeled)	1 small handful of fresh parsley	½ lemon	½ lemon
½ small pineapple	1 large handful of spinach	1 small handful of fresh parsley	2 large handfuls of spinach
1 handful of strawberries		2 large handfuls of spinach	½ avocado
		½ avocado	
- - - - - - - - - - - - - - - - - -	- - - - - - - - - - - - - - - - - -	- - - - - - - - - - - - - - - - - -	- - - - - - - - - - - - - - - - - -
★ Juice all ingredients except the bee pollen and strawberries	★ Juice all ingredients except the flax seed	★ Juice all ingredients except the avocado	★ Juice all ingredients except the avocado
★ Blend with the bee pollen and strawberries until smooth	★ Blend with flax seed, or stir in well	★ Blend with avocado until smooth and creamy	★ Blend with avocado until smooth and creamy

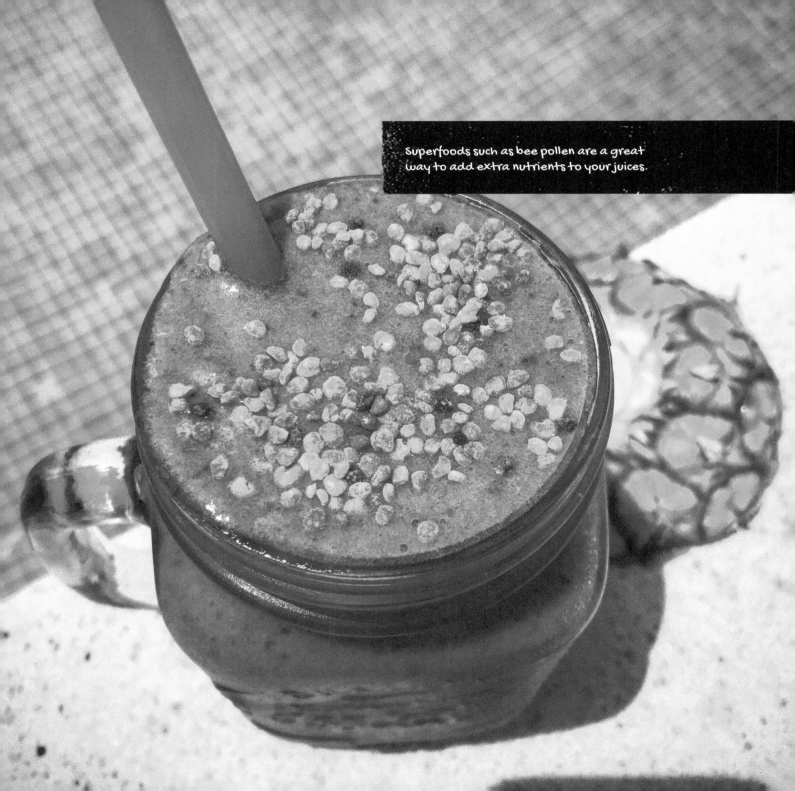

Superfoods such as bee pollen are a great way to add extra nutrients to your juices.

Green Goblin	Greenie Meanie	Immune Booster	Kick Starter
1 broccoli stem	1 broccoli stem	2 apples	1 celery stick
2 celery sticks	2 celery sticks	3 large carrots	½ English cucumber
½ English cucumber	1 English cucumber	½ English cucumber	1 fennel bulb
1 lime (peeled)	1 medium chunk of ginger	1 small chunk of ginger	1 medium chunk of ginger
1 small handful of fresh parsley	1 lime (peeled)	1 lemon	1 lemon
2 tomatoes	3 large handfuls of spinach	1 small handful of fresh parsley	1 large handful of lettuce
½ yellow pepper		1 pear	1 large handful of fresh parsley
½ avocado			
- - - - - - - - - - - - - - - - -	- - - - - - - - - - - - - - - - -	- - - - - - - - - - - - - - - - -	- - - - - - - - - - - - - - - - -
★ Juice all ingredients except the avocado	★ Juice all ingredients	★ Juice all ingredients	★ Juice all ingredients
★ Blend with avocado until smooth and creamy			

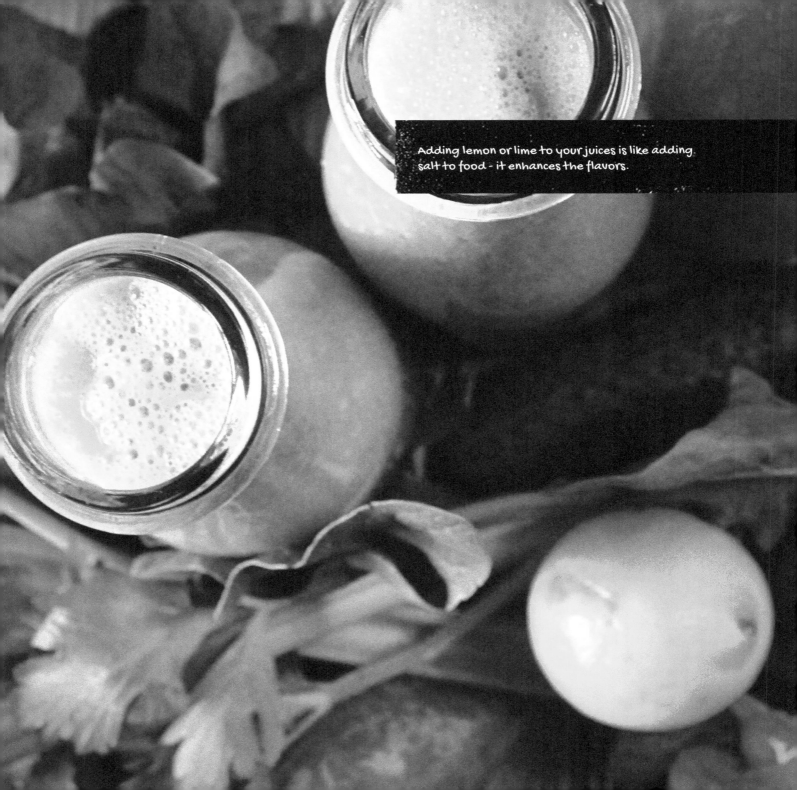

Adding lemon or lime to your juices is like adding salt to food - it enhances the flavors.

Lemon Zing	Mega Mix	Meta Boost	Morning Bliss
1 apple	1 apple	1 beetroot	2 apples
2 carrots	1 beetroot	2 large carrots	1 celery stick
2 celery sticks	1 broccoli stem	2 celery sticks	½ English cucumber
½ English cucumber	1 carrot	½ English cucumber	½ lemon
½ fennel bulb	1 celery stick	1 small chunk of ginger	1 pear
1 small chunk of ginger	½ courgette	½ lemon	1 large handful of spinach
1 lemon	½ English cucumber	1 small handful of fresh parsley	½ avocado
1 small handful of fresh mint	1 small chunk of ginger	2 large handfuls of fresh spinach	
1 small handful of fresh parsley	½ lemon		
½ yellow pepper	1 large handful of spinach		
	½ avocado		

Lemon Zing

★ Juice all ingredients

Mega Mix

★ Juice all ingredients except the avocado

★ Blend with avocado until smooth and creamy

Meta Boost

★ Juice all ingredients

Morning Bliss

★ Juice all ingredients except the avocado

★ Blend with avocado until smooth and creamy

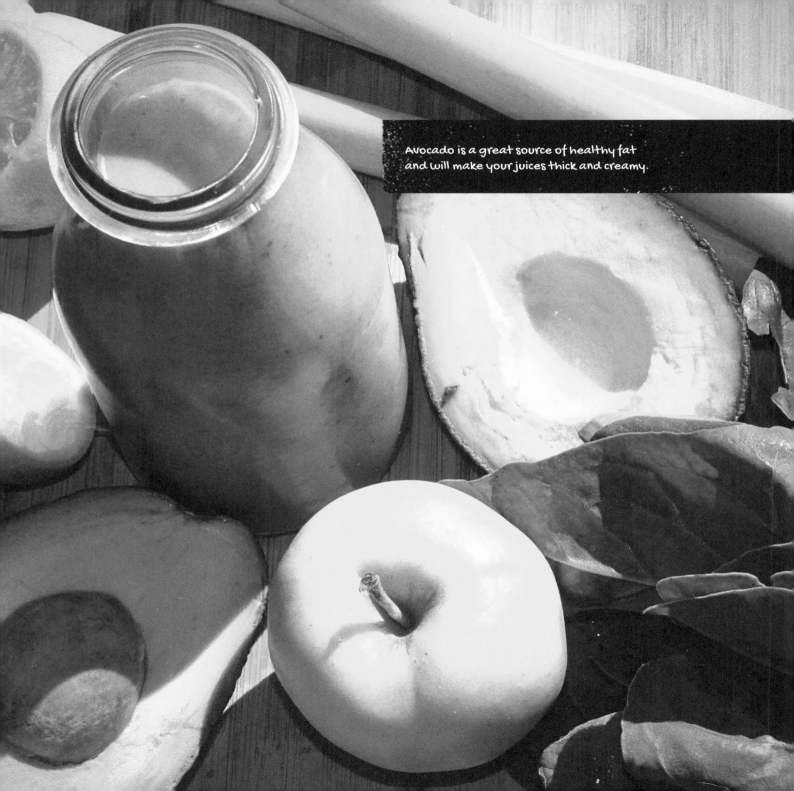

Avocado is a great source of healthy fat and will make your juices thick and creamy.

	P-Arrot	'Pear' Fect	Pharmacia	Pina Coladà

P-Arrot

3 carrots

½ English cucumber

1 small chunk of ginger

½ lemon

1 large orange (peeled)

2 pears

1 small handful of fresh parsley

- - - - - - - - - - - - - - - - - - - -

★ Juice all ingredients

'Pear' Fect

1 celery stick

1 courgette

½ English cucumber

½ lemon

2 pears

1 large handful of spinach

½ avocado

- - - - - - - - - - - - - - - - - - - -

★ Juice all ingredients except the avocado

★ Blend with avocado until smooth and creamy

Pharmacia

1 beetroot

2 carrots

½ English cucumber

1 small chunk of ginger

1 large handful of kale

1 lemon

1 small handful of fresh parsley

1 large handful of spinach

- - - - - - - - - - - - - - - - - - - -

★ Juice all ingredients

Pina Coladà

1 large carrot

1 cup of coconut milk

1 handful of ice

1 lime (peeled)

2 pears

½ small Pineapple

½ avocado

- - - - - - - - - - - - - - - - - - - -

★ Juice all ingredients except the coconut milk, ice, and avocado

★ Blend with coconut milk, ice, and avocado until smooth and creamy

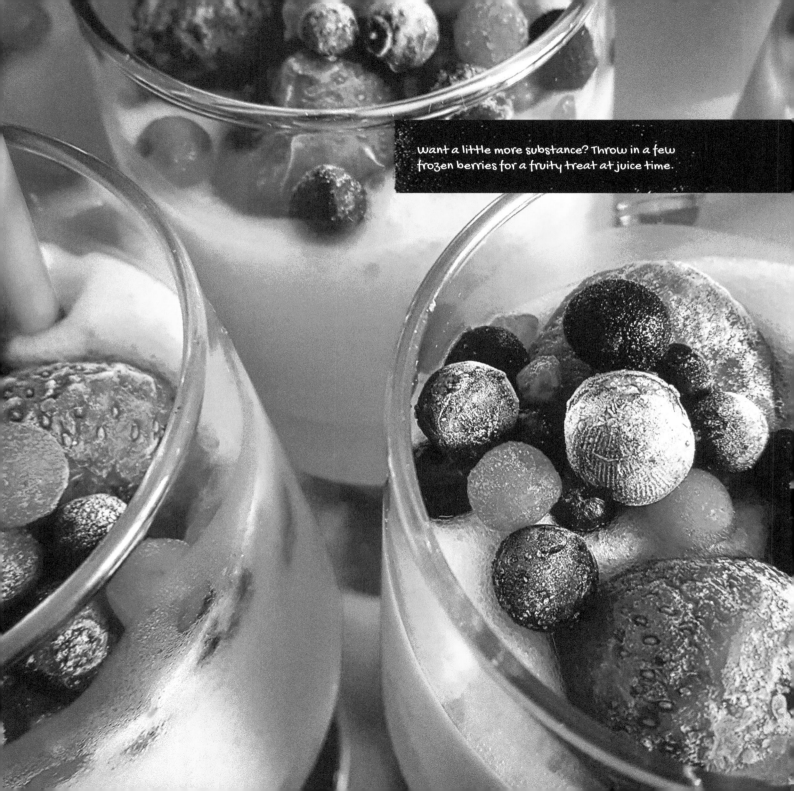

Want a little more substance? Throw in a few frozen berries for a fruity treat at juice time.

Pineapple Kick	Pine Blast	Popeye's Detox	Power Up
1 celery stick	1 cup of coconut milk	2 apples	2 large carrots
½ English cucumber	1 small chunk of ginger (optional)	2 celery sticks	½ English cucumber
1 medium chunk of ginger	1 handful of ice	1 courgette	1 small chunk of ginger
1 lime (peeled)	1 lime (peeled)	1 small chunk of ginger	1 lime (peeled)
2 large oranges (peeled)	1 large orange (peeled)	½ lemon	1 small handful of fresh parsley
½ small pineapple	½ small pineapple	1 small handful of fresh parsley	1 large handful of spinach
--------------------	2 large handfuls of spinach	4 large handfuls of spinach	2 tomatoes
★ Juice all ingredients	--------------------	½ avocado	1 yellow pepper
	★ Juice all ingredients except the coconut milk and ice	--------------------	½ avocado
	★ Blend with the coconut milk and ice until smooth and creamy	★ Juice all ingredients except the avocado	--------------------
		★ Blend with the avocado until smooth and creamy	★ Juice all ingredients except the avocado
			★ Blend with the avocado until smooth and creamy

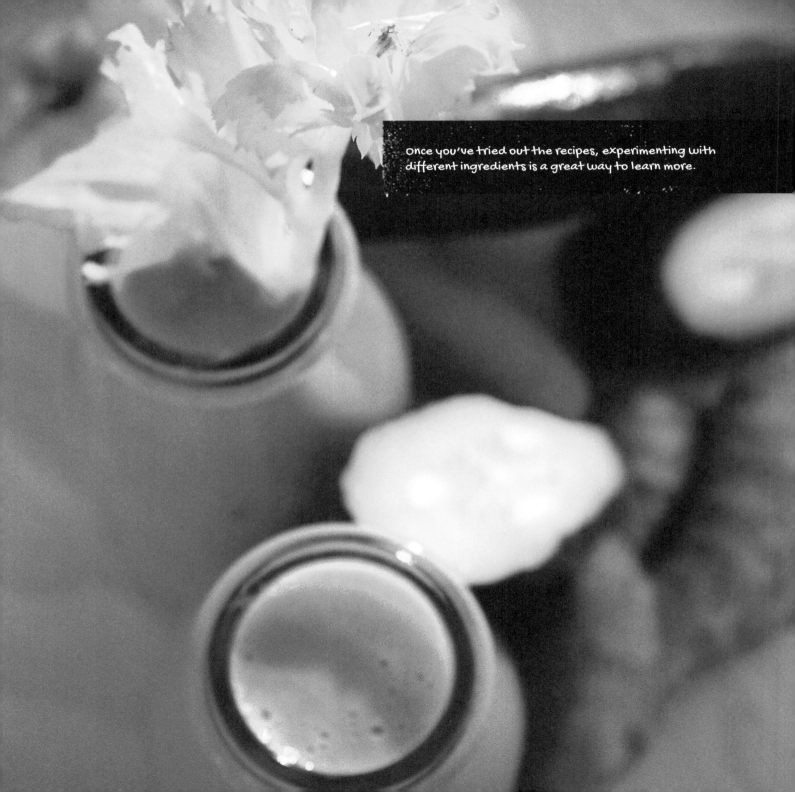

Once you've tried out the recipes, experimenting with different ingredients is a great way to learn more.

Purple Rain	Red Mud	Red Raindrop	Red Robot
2 beetroots	1 apple	1 apple	1 apple
2 large carrots	1 beetroot	1 beetroot	1 beetroot
½ English cucumber	2 carrots	2 celery sticks	2 large carrots
1 lemon	1 courgette	1 fennel bulb	1 small chunk of ginger
1 large handful of lettuce	1 small chunk of ginger	1 lemon	½ lemon
150g red cabbage	½ lemon	1 small handful of fresh parsley	½ avocado
-------------------	1 pear	2 large handfuls of spinach	1 handful of strawberries
★ Juice all ingredients	½ red pepper	-------------------	-------------------
	1 large handful of spinach	★ Juice all ingredients	★ Juice all ingredients except the avocado and strawberries
	½ avocado		★ Blend with the avocado and strawberries until smooth and creamy
	-------------------		
	★ Juice all ingredients except the avocado		
	★ Blend with the avocado until smooth and creamy		

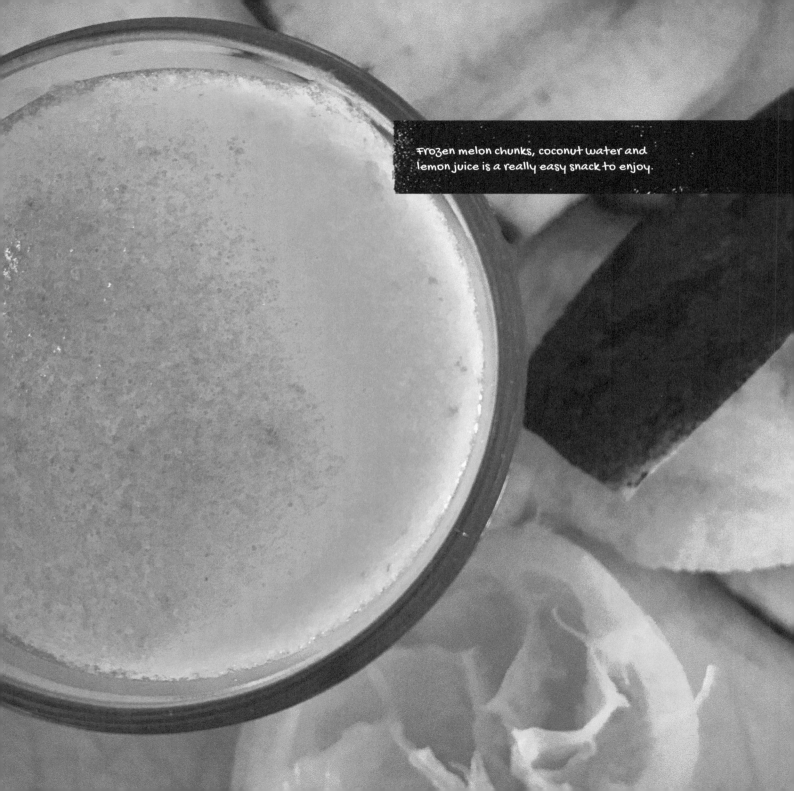

Frozen melon chunks, coconut water and lemon juice is a really easy snack to enjoy.

Salad

2 carrots

1 celery stick

½ English cucumber

1 clove of garlic (optional)

1 lemon

1 large handful of lettuce

pinch of sea salt (optional)

1 tomato

1 yellow pepper

½ avocado

- -

★ Juice all ingredients
  except the avocado,
  garlic, and salt (if using)

★ Blend with the avocado,
  garlic, and salt (if using)
  until smooth and creamy

Sweet Tooth

1 apple

2 carrots

½ English cucumber

1 lemon

1 large handful of lettuce

1 small handful of fresh parsley

½ red pepper

2 tomatoes

½ avocado

- -

★ Juice all ingredients
  except the avocado

★ Blend with the avocado
  until smooth and creamy

Vampire's Dream

2 apples

1 beetroot

3 large carrots

1 celery stick

1 lime (peeled)

½ avocado

- -

★ Juice all ingredients
  except the avocado

★ Blend with the avocado
  until smooth and creamy

Smoothie bowls

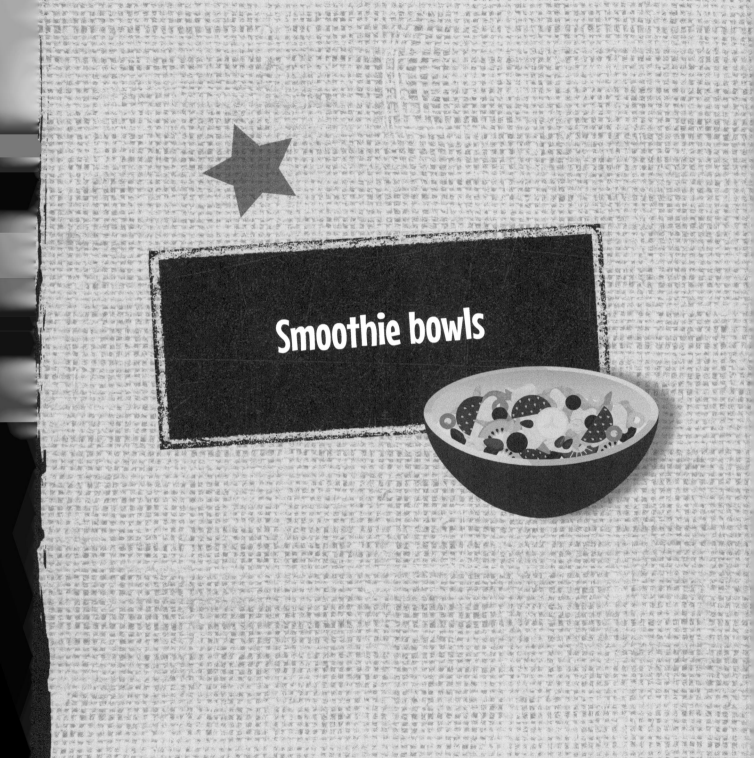

Smoothie bowls are pretty much what they sound like — smoothies in a bowl. They taste great, and are a great way to get some good stuff into you at the start of the day, quickly and easily. With imagination, you can create almost any combination of flavours you want.

These bowls are becoming more and more trendy, and many photo-sharing social media applications have pages dedicated to them. Go take a look!

While measuring quantities is generally a good idea, we like to do things the simpler way. With smoothie bowls, we just measure by the handful. The size of your fist is a good indicator of the quantity of food you can digest comfortably in a single sitting.

To prepare for the week ahead, throw all the ingredients you plan to use into plastic freezer bags and place them in the freezer. This way, when it comes time to make your smoothie bowl, all you need to do is pull out a bag and chuck it in the blender.

Once you've whizzed up your ingredients and they're nice and smooth, pour the mixture into a bowl. Finish by adding the toppings of your choice (we haven't put instructions with each and every recipe, so get creative).

Here's a quick tip — if you're looking to make awesome designs, add the heaviest topping ingredients last.

Please note that each of these recipes makes one serving.

Bana Cado

Ingredients	Toppings
1 frozen banana	1 small handful of D-Toxd C: Real (or granola)
½ avocado	1 tbsp of cacao nibs
1 handful of blueberries	1 tsp of bee pollen
½ cup of almond milk	1 tsp of almond butter
2 handfuls of baby spinach	drizzle of honey

Banana Berry

Ingredients	Toppings
1 frozen banana	sliced banana
1 handful of frozen berries	2 or 3 fresh berries of choice, halved or sliced
1 tbsp of hemp seed	1 tbsp of chia seeds
½ cup of almond milk	1 tbsp of toasted pumpkin seeds
	1 tbsp of desiccated coconut

Banana Split

Ingredients	Toppings
1 frozen banana	2 or 3 fresh strawberries, sliced
1 handful of frozen strawberries	1 tbsp of cacao nibs
½ avocado	1 tbsp of toasted almond flakes
1 small tub of natural yogurt (100g)	2 dates, chopped
½ cup almond milk	drizzle of honey

Prepare your toppings in advance and keep them in an airtight container in the fridge.

Caribbean Bowl

Ingredients	Toppings
1 handful of frozen pineapple	½ peach, sliced
1 frozen banana	1 small handful of blackberries
100ml coconut water	1 tbsp of sunflower seeds
5 mint leaves	2 tbsp of toasted cereal (for crunch)
1 tbsp of honey	drizzle of honey

Courgette and Coconut

Ingredients	Toppings
1 frozen banana	1 handful of blueberries
1 frozen courgette (cut up before freezing)	1 tbsp of pumpkin seeds
½ cup of coconut milk	2 dates, chopped
1 tbsp of almond butter	sliced banana
1 tbsp of chia seeds	1 tbsp of desiccated coconut
½ tsp of cinnamon	1 tsp of hemp seeds

Green Garden

Ingredients	Toppings
1 apple, core removed	2 tbsp of toasted walnuts, chopped
½ avocado	2 tbsp of dried apricots, sliced
1 frozen banana	1 tbsp of cranberries
1 handful of baby spinach	drizzle of honey
½ cup of coconut water	sprinkle of bee pollen
1 tbsp of honey	
juice of 1 lemon	

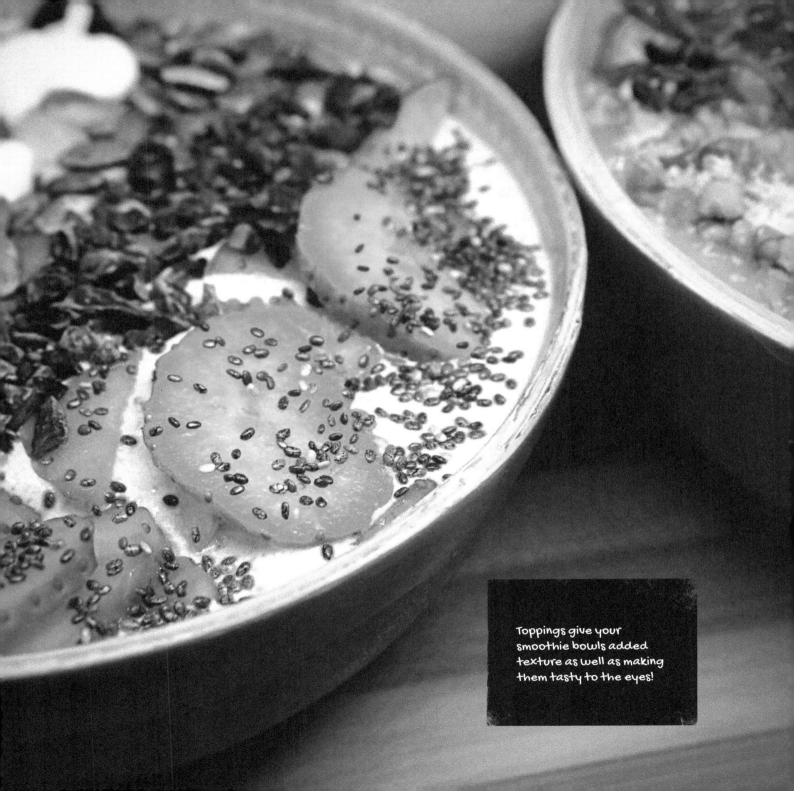

Toppings give your smoothie bowls added texture as well as making them tasty to the eyes!

Mango Delight

Ingredients	Toppings
1 frozen courgette (cut up before freezing)	Fresh mango slices
½ avocado	1 tbsp of toasted almonds or almond flakes
1 handful of baby spinach	fresh blueberries
1 handful of frozen strawberries	1 tbsp of peanut butter
1 handful of frozen mango	drizzle of honey
½ cup of almond milk	
½ cup of ice	

Peanut Butter and Chocolate

Ingredients	Toppings
1 frozen banana	2 tbsp of toasted oats
100ml of almond milk	1 tsp of cacao nibs
3 or 4 ice cubes or frozen strawberries	1 tbsp of toasted almonds or almond flakes
2 tbsp of peanut butter	2 dates, chopped
1 tsp of cacao powder	½ banana, sliced
1 tsp of bee pollen	drizzle of honey
1 tsp of maca powder (optional)	
1 tbsp of honey	

Spinach and Blueberry

Ingredients	Toppings
1 large handful of frozen blueberries	1 small handful of chopped pineapple
½ avocado	1 tbsp of toasted pumpkin seeds
1 frozen banana	1 tbsp of toasted oats
2 handfuls of baby spinach	1 tbsp of almond flakes
½ cup of apple juice	½ tsp of bee pollen
	drizzle of honey

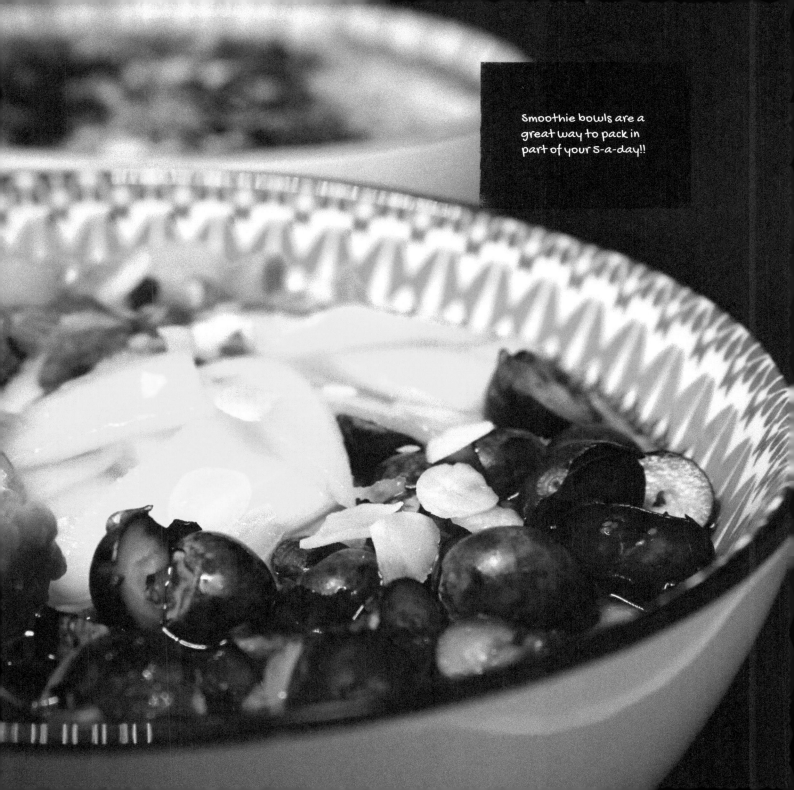

Smoothie bowls are a great way to pack in part of your 5-a-day!!

Tropical Smoothie

Ingredients	Toppings
1 handful of frozen mango	2 or 3 tbsp of chopped fresh mango
1 handful of frozen pineapple	1 kiwi, peeled and sliced
1 banana	2 tbsp of desiccated coconut
½ cup of coconut water	1 tbsp of goji berries
	1 tbsp of walnuts, chopped
	chopped fresh mint (optional)

Vanilla Strawberry

Ingredients	Toppings
1 handful of frozen strawberries	3 or 4 fresh strawberries, sliced
1 small tub of soy or natural yogurt 100g (keep	1 small handful of blueberries
1 tbsp aside for topping)	1 tbsp of toasted almonds, chopped
¼ cup of almond milk	1 tbsp of pumpkin seeds
1 tbsp of honey	1 tsp of chia seeds
½ tsp of vanilla essence	½ tsp of cacao nibs

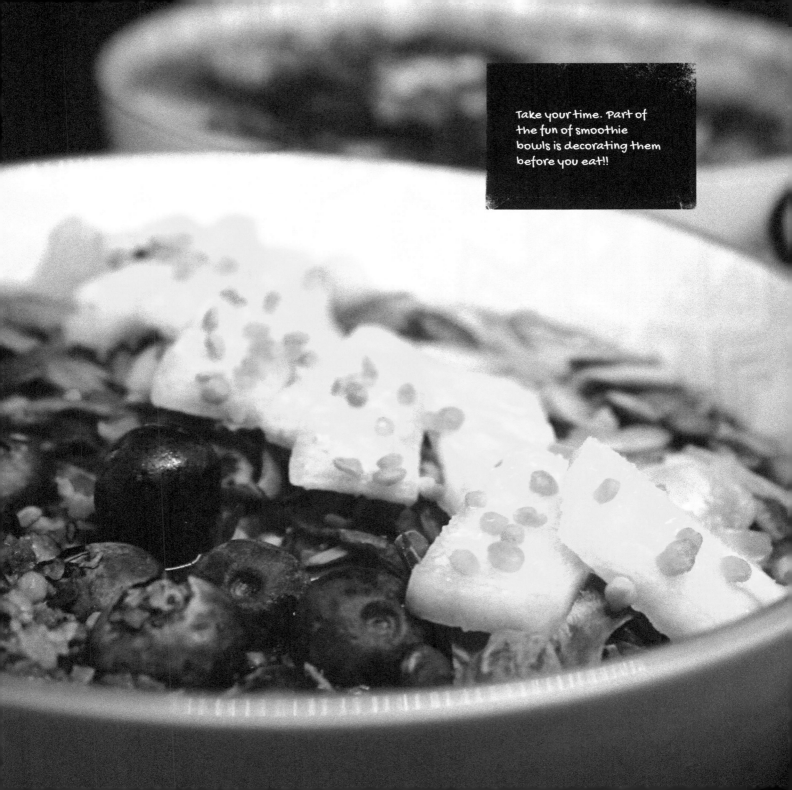

Take your time. Part of the fun of smoothie bowls is decorating them before you eat!!

Breakfasts

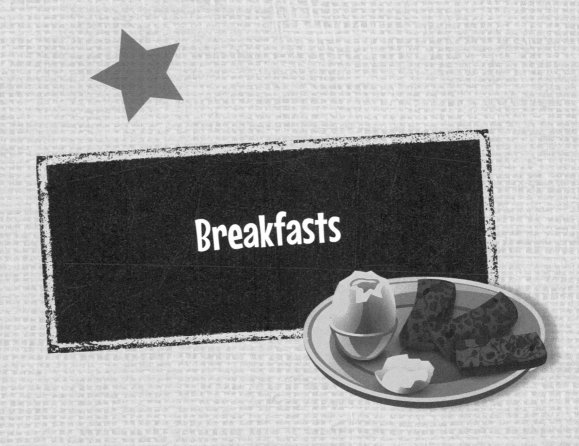

There are times when you want something a little more substantial for breakfast than juices or smoothies. The following is a collection of some of our favourite breakfasts.

Some involve cooking. Some don't. Some need to be prepared the night before. Some don't.

As they say, variety is the spice of life. Why not spice it up?

Breakfast egg muffins

An easy grab and go for those busy mornings, these are protein-packed pockets of good things. They're simple to make and super tasty, too!

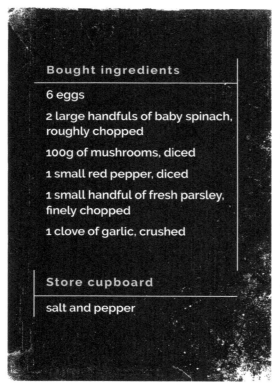

Bought ingredients

6 eggs

2 large handfuls of baby spinach, roughly chopped

100g of mushrooms, diced

1 small red pepper, diced

1 small handful of fresh parsley, finely chopped

1 clove of garlic, crushed

Store cupboard

salt and pepper

Putting it together

★ Preheat oven to 180 degrees Celsius and lightly coat a six-cup muffin tin with cooking spray or line with paper liners.

★ Crack the eggs into a large mixing bowl and whisk until the eggs are smooth.

★ Add the prepared fresh ingredients and stir until everything is well combined.

★ Divide the mixture evenly among the muffin cups, season, and place in the preheated oven.

★ Bake for about fifteen minutes, or until the eggs are set.

★ Serve straight away, or store in the fridge in an airtight container until you're ready to eat them.

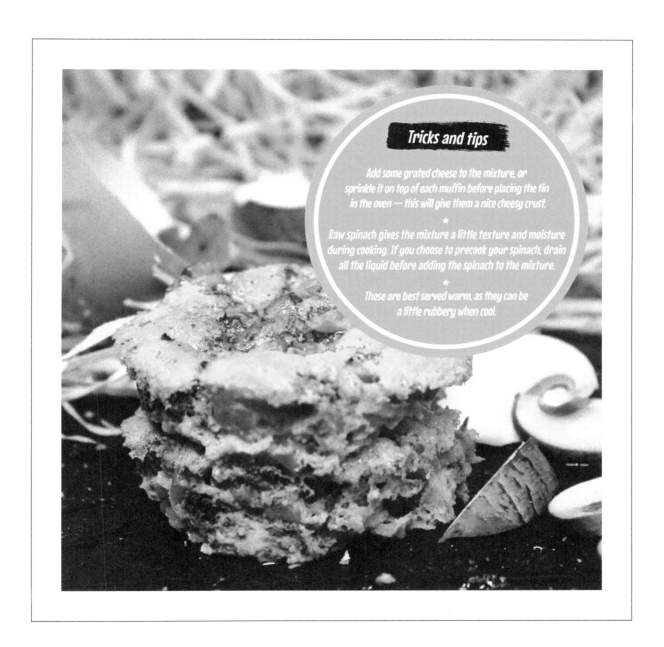

Tricks and tips

Add some grated cheese to the mixture, or sprinkle it on top of each muffin before placing the tin in the oven — this will give them a nice cheesy crust.

★

Raw spinach gives the mixture a little texture and moisture during cooking. If you choose to precook your spinach, drain all the liquid before adding the spinach to the mixture.

★

These are best served warm, as they can be a little rubbery when cool.

Breakfast parfait

A delicious, creamy alternative to a yogurt-based breakfast, this cashew nut cream can be made the night before. Just dish it up in the morning.

Bought ingredients	Store cupboard
125g of cashew nuts	1 tsp of vanilla essence
125ml of coconut milk	
4 or 5 fresh strawberries, sliced	3 tbsp of dried oats
1 banana, sliced	Honey

Putting it together

★ Soak the cashew nuts in water for about thirty minutes, to soften them a little.

★ Place cashew nuts, coconut milk, and vanilla essence in a blender and blend until smooth and creamy.

★ Toast the oats — simply heat up a frying pan, toss the oats in, and stir them around until they start to warm up. They'll start to get dryer, and release a delicious smell, too. Don't leave them for too long, or they'll burn (about four or five minutes is all it takes).

★ In a small glass, layer the cashew cream, sliced fruit, and oats.

★ Drizzle with a bit of honey.

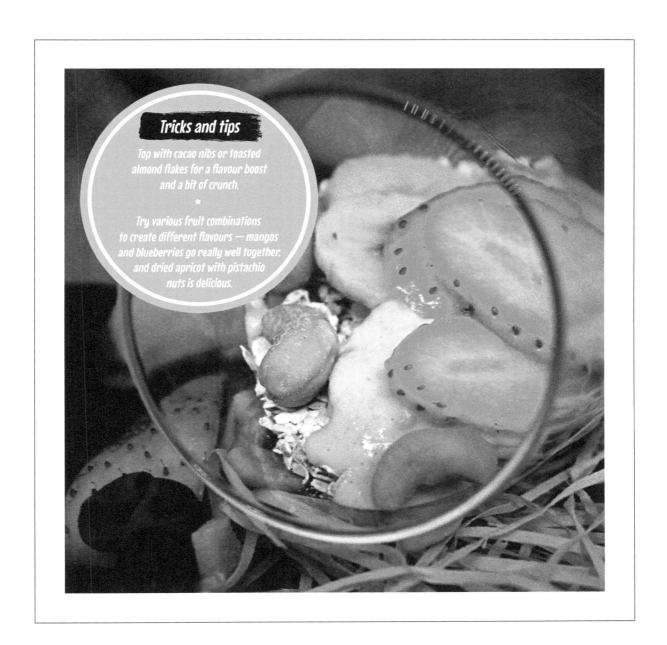

Tricks and tips

Top with cacao nibs or toasted almond flakes for a flavour boost and a bit of crunch.

★

Try various fruit combinations to create different flavours — mangos and blueberries go really well together, and dried apricot with pistachio nuts is delicious.

Breakfast tortilla

Traditionally, the Spanish incorporate potatoes into their tortillas (Spanish omelettes), but we've made some slight alterations.

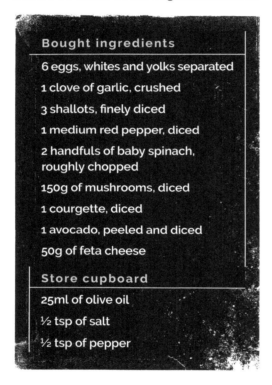

Bought ingredients

6 eggs, whites and yolks separated

1 clove of garlic, crushed

3 shallots, finely diced

1 medium red pepper, diced

2 handfuls of baby spinach, roughly chopped

150g of mushrooms, diced

1 courgette, diced

1 avocado, peeled and diced

50g of feta cheese

Store cupboard

25ml of olive oil

½ tsp of salt

½ tsp of pepper

Putting it together

★ Preheat your oven to 150 degrees Celsius.

★ Separate the yolks from the egg whites. In a large mixing bowl, whisk the egg whites until firm, then set aside.

★ Lightly heat your olive oil in a medium-sized frying pan. Add the garlic, shallots, and red pepper and gently fry until everything is nicely mixed and soft.

★ Add the mushrooms, courgette, and salt and pepper, as well as half the baby spinach, and fry on low heat for a few minutes (don't let the vegetables get too soft).

★ Add the yolks to the beaten egg whites and gently mix them with a wooden spoon. Keep the mixture light and airy.

★ Pour the egg mixture into the frying pan and then shake the pan gently to ensure all the vegetables are coated with the egg.

★ Turn down the heat and leave the pan on the stove for five minutes; the eggs will start to set while cooking. Make sure the heat isn't too high, so the bottom doesn't catch.

★ Once the tortilla has started to firm up, sprinkle the avocado and feta cheese over it and then place the frying pan in the preheated oven, under the grill. This will allow the top of the tortilla to cook. You'll know it's ready when it starts to turn

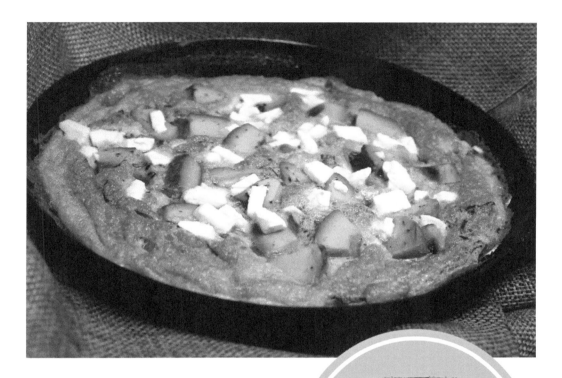

golden brown (this will take about seven or eight minutes on a low to medium heat).

★ Remove from the oven and gently slide the tortilla out of the pan onto a large plate. Cool slightly.

★ Slice into wedges and serve on top of the remaining baby spinach.

Tricks and tips

Add boiled new potatoes instead of courgette (though we find this can be quite heavy for a breakfast).

★

Keep the tortilla in an airtight container and eat it for lunch or dinner with a side of salad.

Breakfast wrap

If you're looking for something different for breakfast, this is ideal!

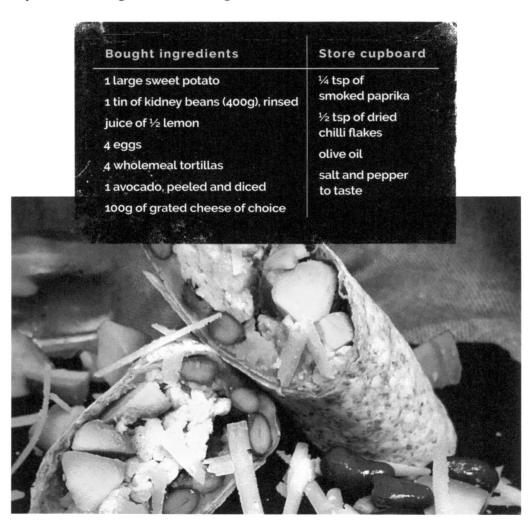

Bought ingredients	Store cupboard
1 large sweet potato	¼ tsp of smoked paprika
1 tin of kidney beans (400g), rinsed	½ tsp of dried chilli flakes
juice of ½ lemon	olive oil
4 eggs	salt and pepper to taste
4 wholemeal tortillas	
1 avocado, peeled and diced	
100g of grated cheese of choice	

Putting it together

★ Preheat your oven to 150 degrees Celsius.

★ Cook the sweet potato in your microwave — pierce the skin a few times with a fork and microwave on high for about five minutes, or until it's cooked through. If you don't use a microwave, you can roast the sweet potato in the oven at about 200 degrees C for thirty minutes.

★ Once the sweet potato is cooked, remove the skin and mash the potato roughly with a fork.

★ In a mixing bowl, combine the drained kidney beans, smoked paprika, dried chilli flakes, and lemon juice and stir.

★ Use the whites of three of the eggs and the whole remaining egg. Whisk the egg whites until they're firm and then, with a wooden spoon, stir in one egg yolk.

★ Drizzle a small amount of olive oil in a frying pan and place on medium heat. Add the egg mixture and cook through, stirring every now and then to create fluffy scrambled eggs (not too much, or they won't be fluffy).

★ Make sure your tortillas are warmed slightly — this will make rolling them easier. Either place them in the microwave for twenty seconds or in a warmed oven for a minute or so.

★ Lay out the tortillas and evenly spread the mashed sweet potato onto each one.

★ Repeat this process with the kidney beans, followed by the avocado, the scrambled eggs, and finally the grated cheese.

★ Season with salt and pepper and then tuck in the ends of the wraps and roll them up.

★ Place the wraps in the preheated oven on a baking tray and let them sit for about five minutes (or until warmed through), to slightly melt the cheese.

★ Enjoy!

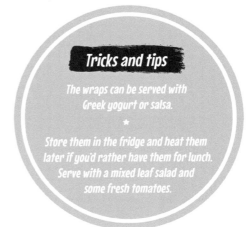

Tricks and tips

The wraps can be served with Greek yogurt or salsa.

★

Store them in the fridge and heat them later if you'd rather have them for lunch. Serve with a mixed leaf salad and some fresh tomatoes.

Chocolate yogurt sundae

A rich, creamy, and refreshing way to start the day.

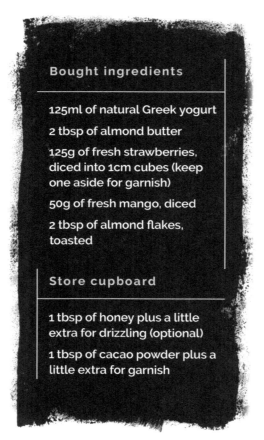

Bought ingredients

125ml of natural Greek yogurt

2 tbsp of almond butter

125g of fresh strawberries, diced into 1cm cubes (keep one aside for garnish)

50g of fresh mango, diced

2 tbsp of almond flakes, toasted

Store cupboard

1 tbsp of honey plus a little extra for drizzling (optional)

1 tbsp of cacao powder plus a little extra for garnish

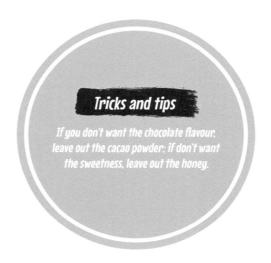

Tricks and tips

If you don't want the chocolate flavour, leave out the cacao powder; if don't want the sweetness, leave out the honey.

Putting it together

★ Place the Greek yogurt, almond butter, honey, and cacao powder in a medium bowl and mix until smooth and creamy.

★ Take two sundae glasses and spoon two tbsp of the chocolate yogurt mix into each of them. Add a layer of chopped strawberries and mango, followed by a layer of almonds.

★ Continue the layering, finishing with the chocolate yogurt.

★ Cut the reserved strawberry in half and place on top of each sundae, followed by a scattering of almonds, a sprinkle of cacao powder, and a drizzle of honey (optional).

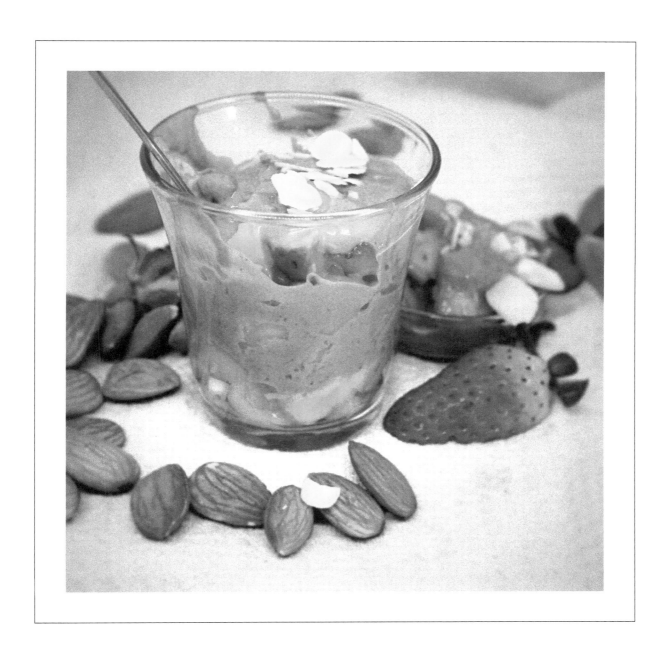

D-Toxd C:Real

There's nothing better than a delicious bowl of cereal in the morning, and once you get the hang of making this one, you'll be set. This recipe makes a big batch. Store it in an airtight container, and it will keep really well for two to three weeks.

Once you have the basic blend, you can add anything you like — we found our favourite combinations by experimenting.

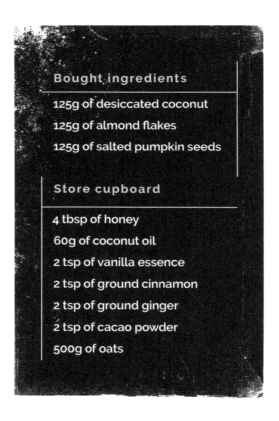

Bought ingredients

125g of desiccated coconut

125g of almond flakes

125g of salted pumpkin seeds

Store cupboard

4 tbsp of honey

60g of coconut oil

2 tsp of vanilla essence

2 tsp of ground cinnamon

2 tsp of ground ginger

2 tsp of cacao powder

500g of oats

Putting it together

★ Place honey and coconut oil into a small pan (or glass container if using your microwave) and heat gently until melted. Stir in vanilla.

★ Preheat your oven to 180 degrees Celsius (or 160 degrees Celsius for fan ovens) and prepare a roasting tray by lining it with greaseproof paper.

★ Place all the remaining ingredients in a large mixing bowl and lightly toss until everything is mixed.

★ Gently pour in the oil mixture and stir. You might want to dive in with your hands and gently rub to give everything a good coating.

★ Pour the mixture into your baking tray, spread it evenly, and place it in the middle of your oven. Leave it to bake for about forty-five minutes, gently mixing it halfway through to ensure it's not burning.

★ Once it's nicely dried out, with a bit of a crunch, remove from the oven and let it cool.

★ Add the fruit of your choice (some examples are provided below), or simply leave it as is and top with fresh fruit and some yogurt or milk of your choice.

Flavour options

★ **Apple and cranberry** — Cut two large apples into quarters (remove the cores), finely slice them, and mix them into your C:Real blend before placing it in the oven, ensuring the apples get nicely mixed in. Once the C:Real has cooled down, add the cranberries.

★ **Dehydrated banana and goji berry** — Once the C:Real has cooled down, mix in 150g of dehydrated banana and 150g of goji berries. We use unsweetened dehydrated banana slices from the local fruit and veg market.

Serving ideas

★ **Greek or soy yogurt** — C:Real is great with yogurt. Place one small tub of unflavoured, unsweetened yogurt in a bowl, sprinkle on

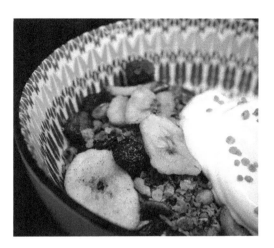

a handful of C:Real, and top with sliced banana.

★ **Yogurt and vanilla soy milk** — This is a good option if you don't like the C:Real too thick. Simply mix one large tbsp of yogurt, a handful of C:Real mix, and a large splash of vanilla soy milk and enjoy.

★ **Bircher C:Real** — Place one large handful of C:Real mix into a bowl, pour on some almond milk (so that it just covers the C:Real) and allow it to stand overnight. Enjoy the following morning, or later in the day as a snack. If the C:Real has thickened too much, add a drop of milk.

Overnight oats

Preparing breakfast the night before always saves you time in the morning, and this creamy oat breakfast will give you the energy you need to power through the day.

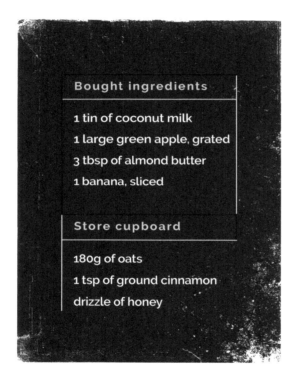

Bought ingredients

1 tin of coconut milk

1 large green apple, grated

3 tbsp of almond butter

1 banana, sliced

Store cupboard

180g of oats

1 tsp of ground cinnamon

drizzle of honey

Putting it together

★ In a bowl, combine the oats, coconut milk, grated apple, and almond butter. Mix well.

★ Cover with cling film and place in the fridge overnight.

★ In the morning, remove from the fridge and stir (it will have thickened overnight). If it's too thick for your liking, add a bit of water or milk to thin it out.

★ Allow it to stand for about fifteen minutes, so that it 'warms up' slightly, or stir through some heated milk to warm it up more if you don't fancy it cold.

★ Garnish with sliced banana, cinnamon, and a drizzle of honey.

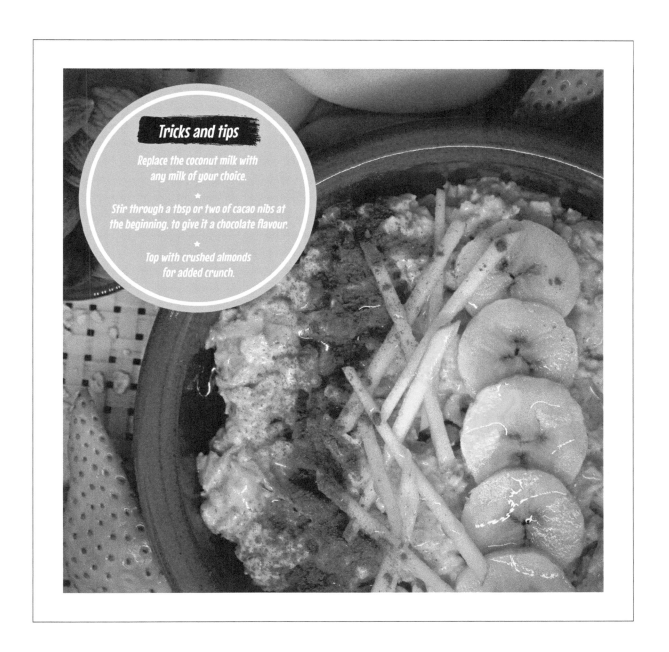

Tricks and tips

Replace the coconut milk with any milk of your choice.

★

Stir through a tbsp or two of cacao nibs at the beginning, to give it a chocolate flavour.

★

Top with crushed almonds for added crunch.

Quinoa chia porridge

A quick and easy breakfast that's prepared the night before, this porridge will save you time in the morning — simply sit down and enjoy it. Chia seeds are said to be one the healthiest foods on the planet, loaded with nutrients for your body and brain, and quinoa is a protein-packed, wheat-free alternative to oats.

Bought ingredients	Store cupboard
3 dates, pitted	125g of cooked quinoa
5 large strawberries, 3 whole, 2 sliced	4 tbsp of chia seeds
200ml of almond milk	
25g of almonds, roughly crushed	
25g of desiccated coconut	

Putting it together

★ Prepare the quinoa by following the directions on the package, and leave to cool.

★ In a blender, add the dates, three strawberries, and almond milk and blend until smooth.

★ Pour into a bowl and add the chia seeds. Mix well, until all the seeds are covered with the liquid and a 'porridge' is created.

Cover with cling film and place in the fridge overnight — the mixture will form a jelly-like substance, so don't panic when you see it.

★ In the morning, place the mixture into a larger bowl, stir in the quinoa, crushed almonds, and coconut and garnish with the remaining strawberries.

★ If you find the porridge is a little thick, you can add a bit more almond milk to thin it out.

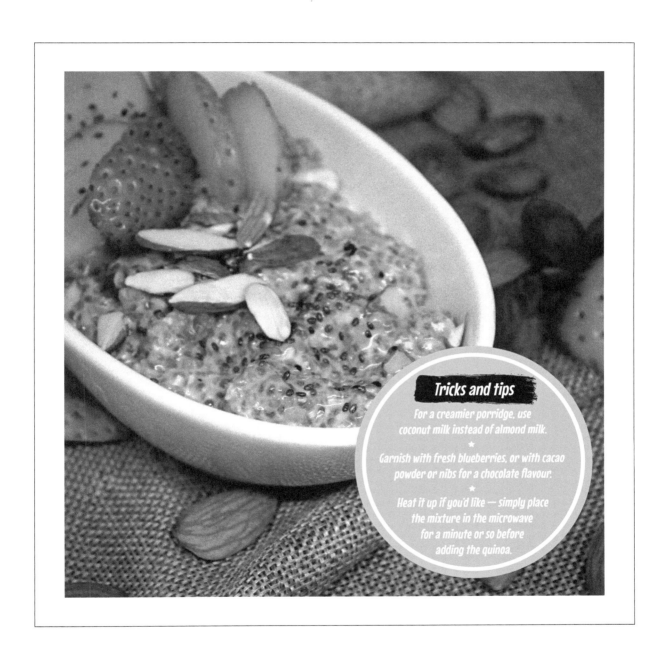

Tricks and tips

For a creamier porridge, use coconut milk instead of almond milk.

★

Garnish with fresh blueberries, or with cacao powder or nibs for a chocolate flavour.

★

Heat it up if you'd like — simply place the mixture in the microwave for a minute or so before adding the quinoa.

Quinoa fruit bowl

Many people think of quinoa as simply a great substitute for rice, but it's much more versatile than that!

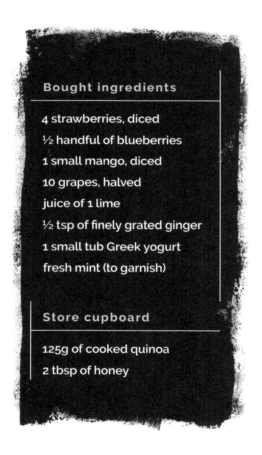

Bought ingredients

4 strawberries, diced

½ handful of blueberries

1 small mango, diced

10 grapes, halved

juice of 1 lime

½ tsp of finely grated ginger

1 small tub Greek yogurt

fresh mint (to garnish)

Store cupboard

125g of cooked quinoa

2 tbsp of honey

Putting it together

★ Prepare the quinoa by following the directions on the package, and leave to cool (you can do this the night before, to save time in the morning).

★ In a bowl, gently toss the quinoa with the chopped fruit until nicely mixed.

★ In a small bowl, mix the lime juice, grated ginger, and honey until well blended.

★ Drizzle the dressing over your quinoa and fruit mixture and toss it until everything is lightly coated.

★ Place yogurt in a serving bowl and spoon over the quinoa and fruit mixture.

★ Garnish with chopped mint and enjoy.

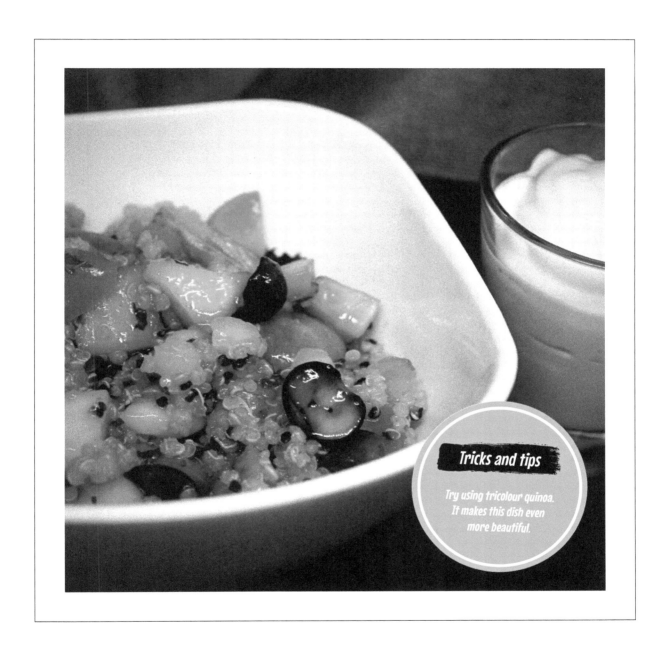

Tricks and tips

Try using tricolour quinoa. It makes this dish even more beautiful.

Scrambled tofu

A tasty alternative to scrambled eggs — and if you make a little extra, it's great with salad.

Bought ingredients	Store cupboard
2 spring onions, sliced	20 ml of olive oil
1 clove of garlic, finely diced	¼ tsp of turmeric
200g of silken tofu, drained	¼ tsp of curry powder or chilli flakes
1 tomato, diced	
1 carrot, peeled and grated	
100g of fresh spinach, finely chopped	½ tsp of salt
squeeze of lemon juice	¼ tsp of pepper

Putting it together

★ Lightly heat the olive oil in a large frying pan and gently fry the onions, garlic, and spices (for two to three minutes only).

★ Roughly chop up the tofu to desired size and toss into the mixture. Fry until golden brown and covered with the onions, garlic, and spices.

★ Mix in the tomato and grated carrot and mix. Don't cook the tomato and carrot — just heat them through.

★ Remove from heat, stir through the spinach, and season to taste.

★ Drizzle with a squeeze of lemon juice and olive oil and serve.

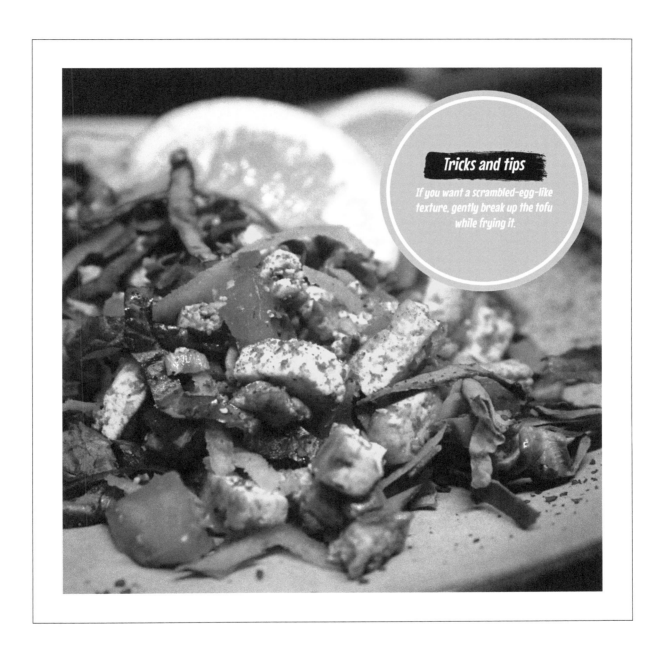

Tricks and tips

If you want a scrambled-egg-like texture, gently break up the tofu while frying it.

Seed cereal

A delicious, wheat-free alternative to granola, this cereal can keep for up to two weeks in an airtight container. This recipe will give you a batch of about eight servings.

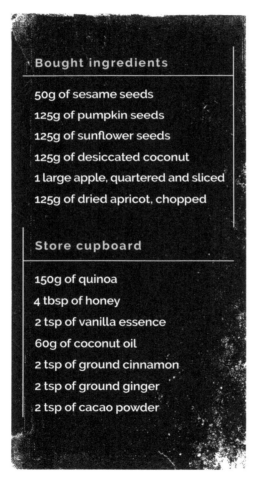

Bought ingredients

50g of sesame seeds

125g of pumpkin seeds

125g of sunflower seeds

125g of desiccated coconut

1 large apple, quartered and sliced

125g of dried apricot, chopped

Store cupboard

150g of quinoa

4 tbsp of honey

2 tsp of vanilla essence

60g of coconut oil

2 tsp of ground cinnamon

2 tsp of ground ginger

2 tsp of cacao powder

Putting it together

★ In a small cup, lightly heat the honey, vanilla, and coconut oil and mix until blended.

★ Preheat your oven to 180 degrees Celsius and prepare a roasting tray by lining it with greaseproof paper.

★ Place the quinoa (cooked per the package's instructions and then cooled), seeds, desiccated coconut, diced apple, and spices in a large mixing bowl. Lightly toss everything until it's all mixed.

★ Gently pour in the oil mixture and stir. You might want to dive in with your hands and gently rub to give everything a good coating.

★ Pour the mixture into your baking tray, spread it evenly, and place it in the middle of your oven. Leave it to bake for about forty-five minutes, gently mixing it halfway through to ensure it's not burning.

★ Once it's nicely dried out, with a bit of a crunch, remove from the oven and let it cool down.

★ Stir through the dried apricot and top with fruit and yogurt or milk of your choice.

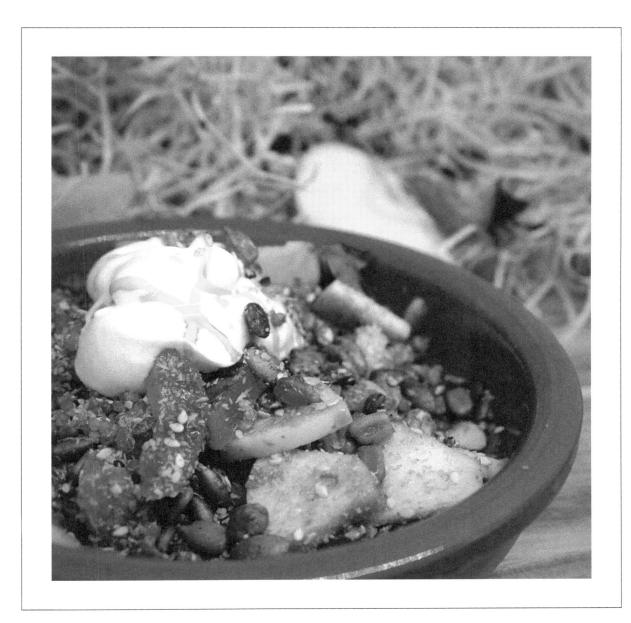

Smoked salmon on toast

This one is so simple it almost doesn't need a recipe, but sometimes people just need a guiding hand to show them how easy a meal can really be.

Bought ingredients	Store cupboard
2 slices of rye bread	salt and pepper
1 tbsp of capers, roughly chopped	
½ small tub of Greek yogurt	
squeeze of lemon juice	
1 small handful of cress	
100g of smoked salmon	
½ red onion, finely sliced	

Putting it together

★ Toast the bread until warm.

★ Mix the capers, yogurt, and lemon juice until well combined.

★ Spread the yogurt mixture onto the slices of toast.

★ Place the cress on top of the yogurt mixture.

★ Layer on the smoked salmon.

★ Sprinkle the sliced onion on top and season to taste.

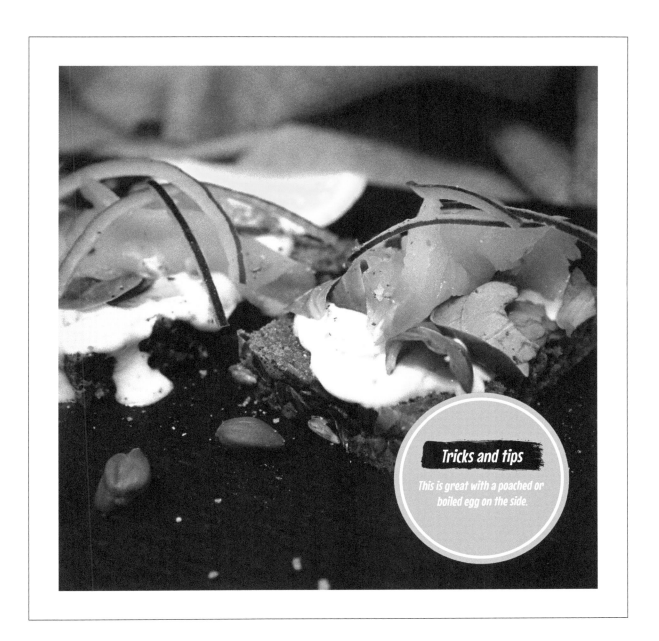

Tricks and tips

This is great with a poached or boiled egg on the side.

Spanish pepper, spinach, and feta tortilla

This tortilla (Spanish omelette) is great for any meal.

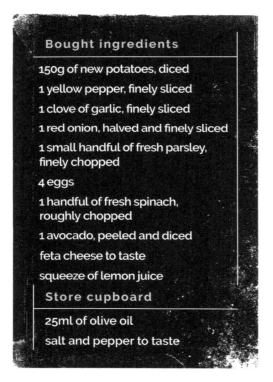

Bought ingredients

150g of new potatoes, diced

1 yellow pepper, finely sliced

1 clove of garlic, finely sliced

1 red onion, halved and finely sliced

1 small handful of fresh parsley, finely chopped

4 eggs

1 handful of fresh spinach, roughly chopped

1 avocado, peeled and diced

feta cheese to taste

squeeze of lemon juice

Store cupboard

25ml of olive oil

salt and pepper to taste

Putting it together

★ In a saucepan, lightly boil the potatoes until they are almost cooked — you want them to be tender but not so cooked that they start to fall apart.

★ In a frying pan, heat half the oil and fry the pepper, garlic, and onion on high heat, stirring well until everything starts to brown slightly. The trick is to stir constantly so that the ingredients don't catch (frying is quicker than roasting and results in a similar flavour).

★ Reduce the heat by half and add the remaining oil, the parsley, and the boiled potatoes and stir until well blended.

★ Separate the whites from two eggs. In a mixing bowl, beat the whites until they start to firm up. You want them well beaten but not too stiff. Add the other two eggs (both whites and yolks) and fold them through the mixture.

★ Pour into the frying pan, add the spinach and avocado, and mix until everything is coated with the egg mixture and nicely blended.

★ Cook gently on low heat for about five minutes (until the tortilla is golden and set underneath).

★ Sprinkle over the feta cheese (to taste) and place under a hot grill until the tortilla is set and golden brown on the top.

★ Slide out of the pan, squeeze over the lemon juice, and let stand for a few minutes.

★ Cut into wedges, season to taste, and enjoy with salad.

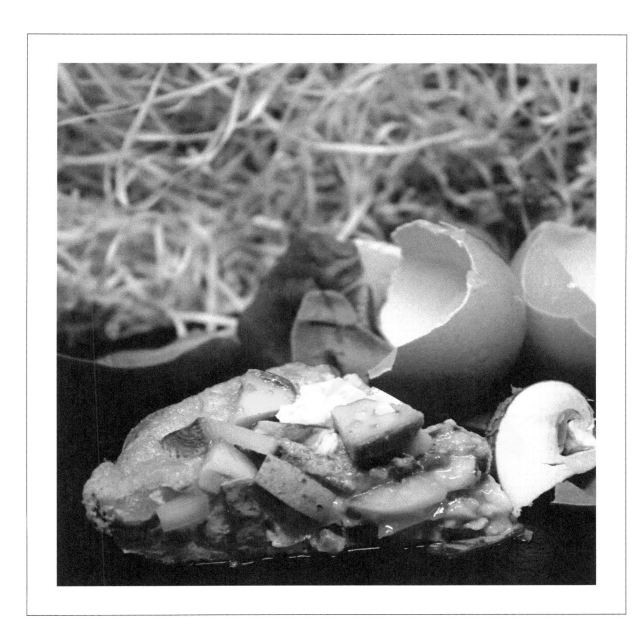

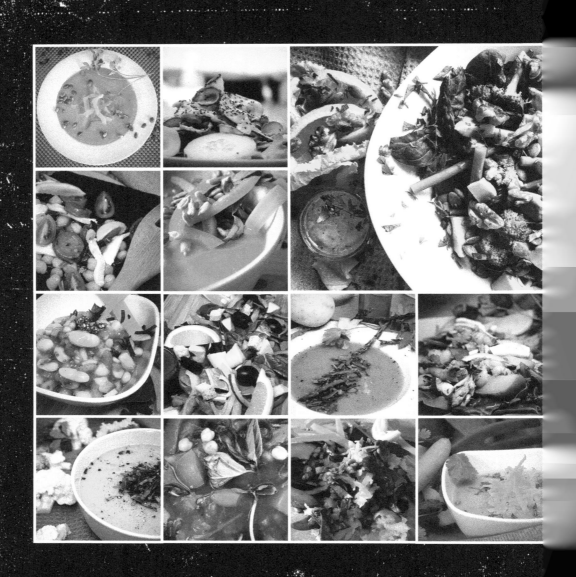

FUEL TO GO:
SALADS AND SOUPS

If you're anything like us, you're constantly juggling tasks, then there is one very precious commodity: time! We all know how important it is to provide the body with the right fuel, but sometimes, time just isn't on our side.

That's why we've created meals you can prepare in advance. With pre-prepared meals, you know you're going to get what you need. After all, if you were going on a long journey, you'd make sure the fuel tank was full, wouldn't you?

Soups are great to batch cook and put in the freezer, and salads are simple and easy to throw together the night before. If you don't want your salads too soggy the next day, simply prepare all the ingredients and store them in separate containers — when you're ready to go, just bosh them all together!

Recipes in this section

SALADS	SOUPS
Apple and carrot spinach slaw	Carrot and coriander soup
Avocado, asparagus, and broccoli salad	Carrot and red pepper soup
Chickpea, avocado, and feta salad	Cauli-broc mustard soup
Courgette with creamy avocado mustard dressing	Chilli butternut squash and ginger soup
D-Toxd baked beans	Chilli chickpea and lemon soup
Mandi's warm mackerel and cannellini bean salad	Courgette, carrot, and sweet potato soup
Miripiri's warm chickpea and chorizo salad	Courgette, pea, and cannellini bean soup
Spinach, avocado, and pepper salad	Courgette, pea, and mint soup
Tomato and chickpea salad	D-Toxd vegetable soup
	Detox super food green vegetable soup
	Leek, asparagus, and baby potato soup
	Potato, asparagus, pea, and mint soup
	Roast red pepper and tomato soup
	Roast tomato and basil soup
	Spicy sweet potato soup

Salads

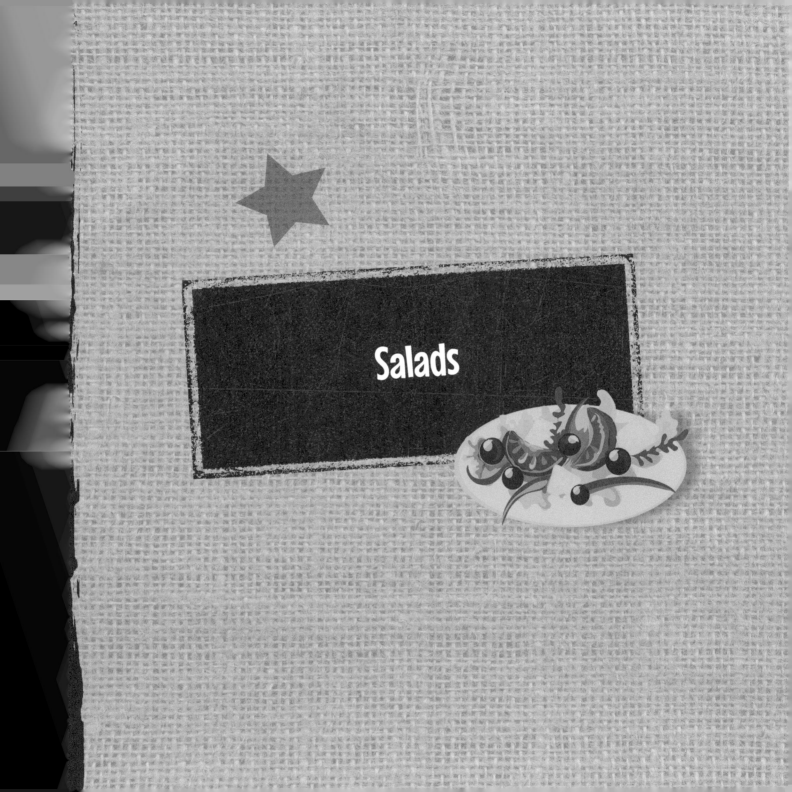

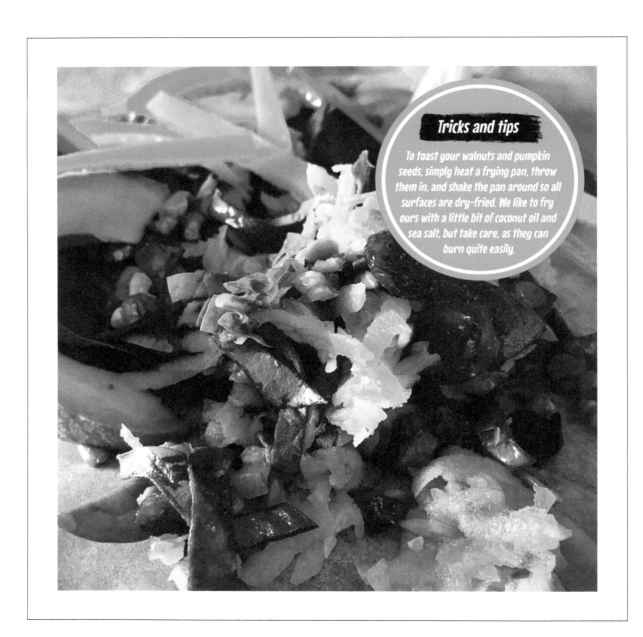

Tricks and tips

To toast your walnuts and pumpkin seeds, simply heat a frying pan, throw them in, and shake the pan around so all surfaces are dry-fried. We like to fry ours with a little bit of coconut oil and sea salt, but take care, as they can burn quite easily.

Apple and carrot spinach slaw

This slightly different take on traditional coleslaw is a refreshing meal on its own and also a delicious side.

Bought ingredients	Store cupboard
juice of 1 lemon	25ml of olive oil
1 avocado, peeled	25ml of apple cider vinegar
1 apple, cored and grated	salt and pepper to taste
1 large carrot, peeled and grated	
1 handful of baby spinach, roughly chopped	
75g of toasted walnuts	
50g of raisins	
25g of toasted sunflower seeds	

Putting it together

★ In a blender, combine the olive oil, vinegar, lemon juice, and avocado until smooth.

★ Place the remaining ingredients in a large bowl and toss until well mixed.

★ Pour over the avocado dressing, mix well, season to taste, and sprinkle over the toasted sunflower seeds.

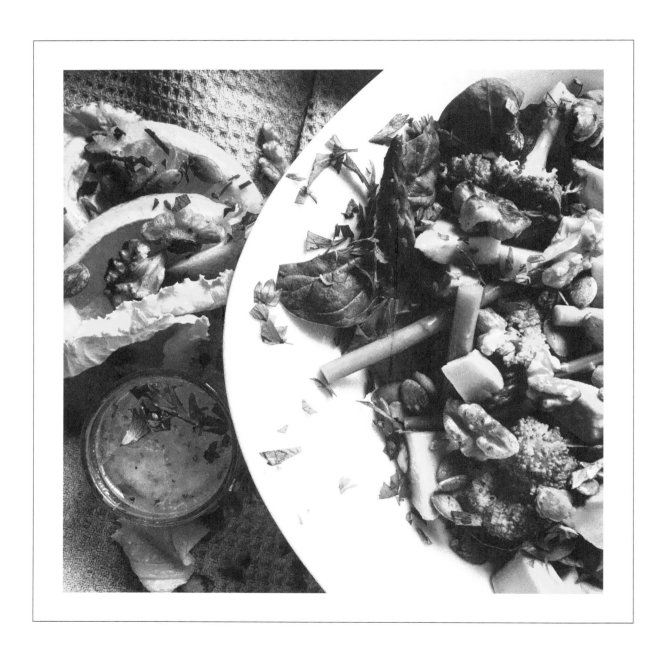

Avocado, asparagus, and broccoli salad

This salad will be a hit during the summer. It's bright, green, full of goodness, and, as Joe Wicks likes to say, 'midget trees'!

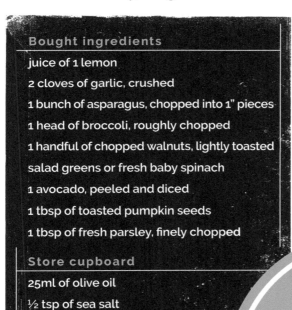

Bought ingredients

juice of 1 lemon

2 cloves of garlic, crushed

1 bunch of asparagus, chopped into 1" pieces

1 head of broccoli, roughly chopped

1 handful of chopped walnuts, lightly toasted

salad greens or fresh baby spinach

1 avocado, peeled and diced

1 tbsp of toasted pumpkin seeds

1 tbsp of fresh parsley, finely chopped

Store cupboard

25ml of olive oil

½ tsp of sea salt

black pepper to taste

★ Lightly steam the asparagus and broccoli until just cooked — you want them to keep their crunch, so steam them for just a few minutes.

★ Place in a large bowl and pour over the dressing, tossing gently to mix the ingredients well.

★ Serve on top of a bed of salad greens or fresh spinach and garnish with avocado, toasted walnuts, pumpkin seeds, and parsley.

Putting it together

★ To prepare the dressing, combine the olive oil, sea salt, lemon juice, and garlic in a container and shake until well mixed. You can also put these ingredients in a small bowl and mix with a fork.

Tricks and tips

Mix all the ingredients in a large bowl before serving — this way, everything gets lightly coated with the refreshing dressing.

★

Black olives go great with this salad, and add a bit of taste and colour.

★

To toast your walnuts and pumpkin seeds, simply heat a frying pan, throw them in, and shake the pan around so all surfaces are dry-fried. We like to fry ours with a little bit of coconut oil and sea salt, but take care, as they can burn quite easily.

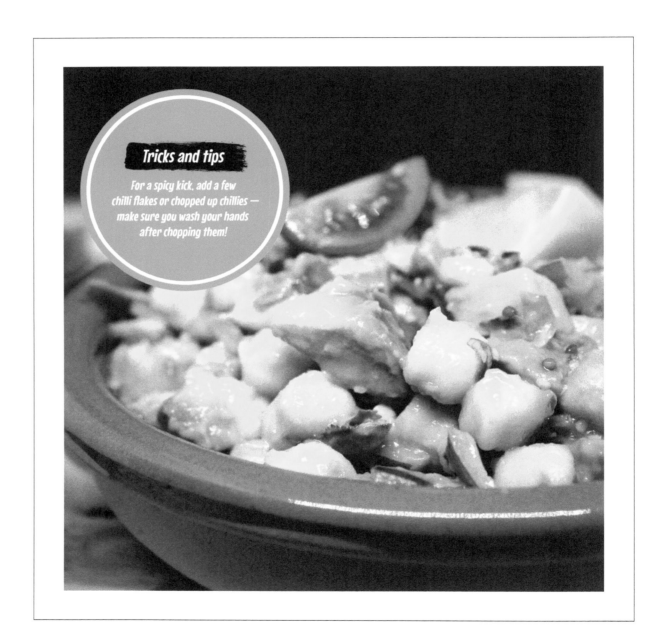

Tricks and tips

For a spicy kick, add a few chilli flakes or chopped up chillies — make sure you wash your hands after chopping them!

Chickpea, avocado, and feta salad

A quick and easy salad for a warm summer evening (or a simple lunch), this is a great source of healthy protein.

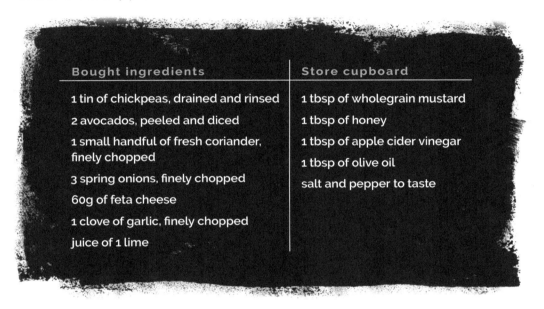

Bought ingredients	Store cupboard
1 tin of chickpeas, drained and rinsed	1 tbsp of wholegrain mustard
2 avocados, peeled and diced	1 tbsp of honey
1 small handful of fresh coriander, finely chopped	1 tbsp of apple cider vinegar
3 spring onions, finely chopped	1 tbsp of olive oil
60g of feta cheese	salt and pepper to taste
1 clove of garlic, finely chopped	
juice of 1 lime	

Putting it together

★ In a medium bowl, combine chickpeas, avocados, coriander, spring onions, feta cheese, and garlic. Toss gently until mixed.

★ In a small bowl, combine the lime juice, mustard, honey, apple cider vinegar, and olive oil and whisk until well blended.

★ Pour over the chickpea mixture and toss so that everything is nicely coated with the dressing.

★ Season with salt and pepper.

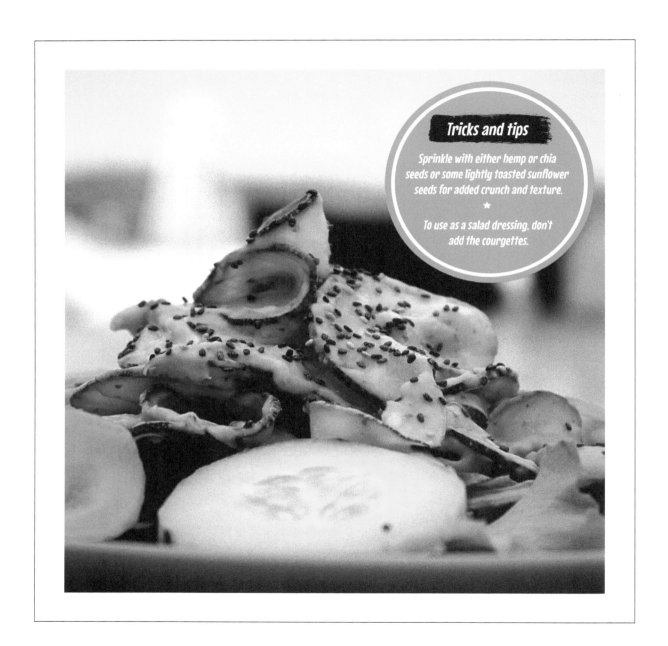

Tricks and tips

Sprinkle with either hemp or chia seeds or some lightly toasted sunflower seeds for added crunch and texture.

★

To use as a salad dressing, don't add the courgettes.

Courgette with creamy avocado mustard dressing

Creamy and refreshing, this dressing is a great addition to salads and can even be eaten on its own.

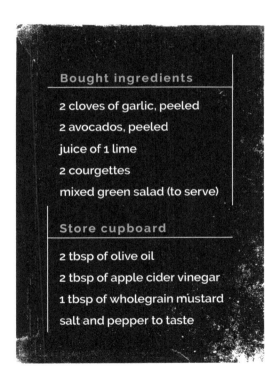

Bought ingredients

2 cloves of garlic, peeled

2 avocados, peeled

juice of 1 lime

2 courgettes

mixed green salad (to serve)

Store cupboard

2 tbsp of olive oil

2 tbsp of apple cider vinegar

1 tbsp of wholegrain mustard

salt and pepper to taste

Putting it together

★ Place garlic, avocados, lime juice, olive oil, and vinegar in a blender and blend until smooth. If the mixture is too thick, add a little water. Remove from the blender and stir through the wholegrain mustard.

★ Peel the courgettes with a potato peeler (lengthways from top to bottom) to create thin, flat ribbons. To get even-sized ribbons, rotate the courgette after three or four peels.

★ Pour the mixture over the courgette ribbons and mix gently until well covered.

★ Season to taste and serve with a mixed green salad.

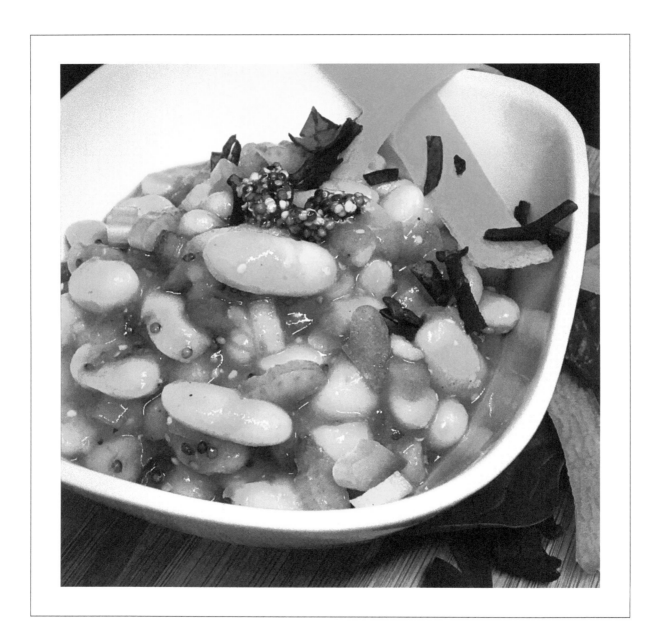

D-Toxd baked beans

These are a great source of protein, a 'meaty' addition to salads, and ideal for a quick snack when you're on the run — this recipe is nearly as easy as opening up a tin of beans.

Bought ingredients	Store cupboard
juice of 1 lemon	1 tsp of honey
1 tin of white beans of choice, drained and rinsed	1 tsp of wholegrain mustard
1 stick of celery, finely diced	1 tbsp of tomato puree
	salt and pepper to taste

Putting it together

★ In a bowl, mix the lemon juice, honey, mustard, and tomato puree until nicely blended.

★ Rinse the beans, place them and the celery in the bowl, and mix well.

★ Season to taste.

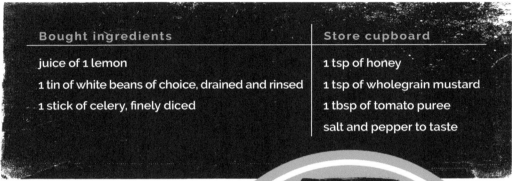

Tricks and tips

For added sweetness, mix in a grated carrot or beetroot (this will also give you a complete meal).

★

Serve on rye bread as a healthy alternative to beans on toast: instead of butter, use home-made hummus.

★

For a more accurate representation of tinned baked beans, add a little water to the mixture to thin it out.

★

Make sure the beans aren't too firm — some tinned varieties can be a bit tough.

★

Serve in a wholemeal wrap with some baby spinach, cucumber, and finely sliced peppers.

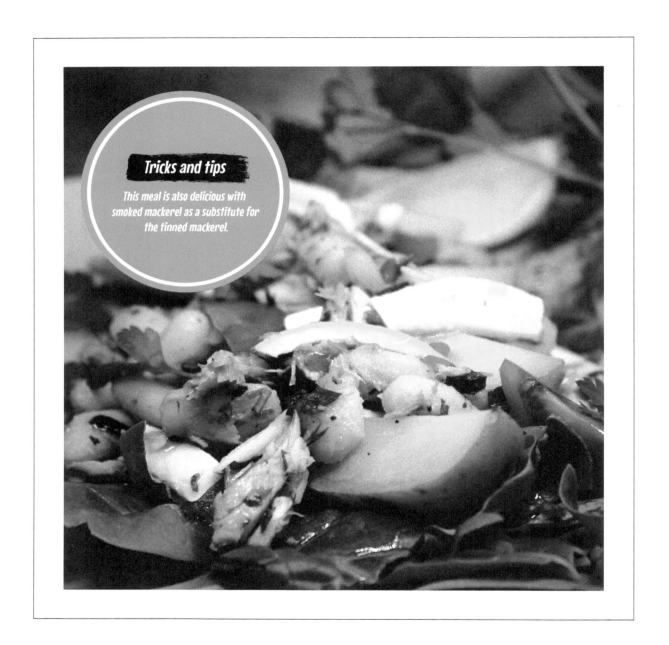

Tricks and tips

This meal is also delicious with smoked mackerel as a substitute for the tinned mackerel.

Mandi's warm mackerel and cannellini bean salad

At the end of the day, sometimes you just want something quick and healthy to eat. This dish is no fuss.

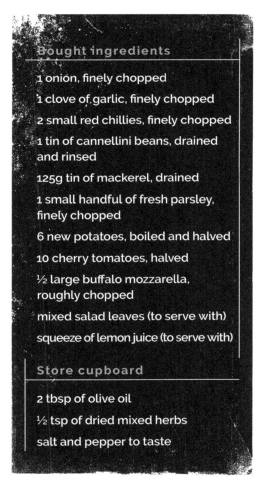

Bought ingredients

1 onion, finely chopped

1 clove of garlic, finely chopped

2 small red chillies, finely chopped

1 tin of cannellini beans, drained and rinsed

125g tin of mackerel, drained

1 small handful of fresh parsley, finely chopped

6 new potatoes, boiled and halved

10 cherry tomatoes, halved

½ large buffalo mozzarella, roughly chopped

mixed salad leaves (to serve with)

squeeze of lemon juice (to serve with)

Store cupboard

2 tbsp of olive oil

½ tsp of dried mixed herbs

salt and pepper to taste

Putting it together

★ Lightly heat the oil in a pot and gently fry the onion, garlic, chillies, and mixed herbs for one minute (until onions are soft and golden brown).

★ Throw in the cannellini beans and stir gently for two to three minutes.

★ Flake up the mackerel, add to the pot and cook for two minutes. If the mixture gets a little thick, add some water (be careful not to stir too much or you'll turn the fish to mush).

★ Remove from heat, stir through the fresh parsley, and let stand for about ten minutes so that it cools down slightly; keep the pot covered with the lid.

★ Boil the new potatoes until soft and tender and cut in half (they'll take about ten to twelve minutes to cook, depending on size).

★ Add the new potatoes, cherry tomatoes, and cheese to the mixture and stir gently, allowing the mozzarella to soften and melt a little.

★ Season to taste and serve with mixed salad leaves and a squeeze of lemon juice.

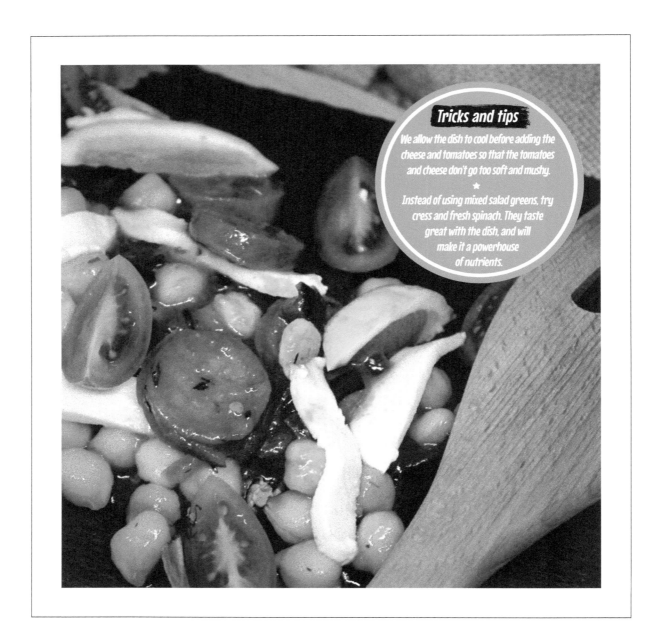

Tricks and tips

We allow the dish to cool before adding the cheese and tomatoes so that the tomatoes and cheese don't go too soft and mushy.

★

Instead of using mixed salad greens, try cress and fresh spinach. They taste great with the dish, and will make it a powerhouse of nutrients.

Miripiri's warm chickpea and chorizo salad

This dish was created using leftover ingredients in the fridge and pantry — it's easy to make and has a great flavour. It was kindly contributed by a close friend of D-Toxd.

Bought ingredients	Store cupboard
1 onion, finely chopped	1 tbsp of olive oil
2 cloves of garlic, finely chopped	2 tsp of dried thyme
1 chorizo sausage, sliced	1 tbsp of honey
100ml of tomato passata	
1 small chilli, finely sliced	
1 tin of chickpeas, drained and rinsed	
½ buffalo mozzarella, roughly chopped or sliced	
1 handful of cherry tomatoes, halved	
mixed salad greens	
juice of 1 lemon	

Putting it together

* Lightly heat the olive oil in a frying pan and gently cook the onion, garlic, chorizo, and thyme until the onion is soft and the chorizo starts to colour the ingredients.

* Pour in the tomato passata and bring to a boil.

* Reduce the heat and add the honey, chilli, and chickpeas; let simmer for three to four minutes on low heat.

* Remove from heat and let cool slightly.

* Stir.

* Add the mozzarella and tomatoes, season to taste, and serve warm on a bed of mixed salad greens with a squeeze of lemon juice.

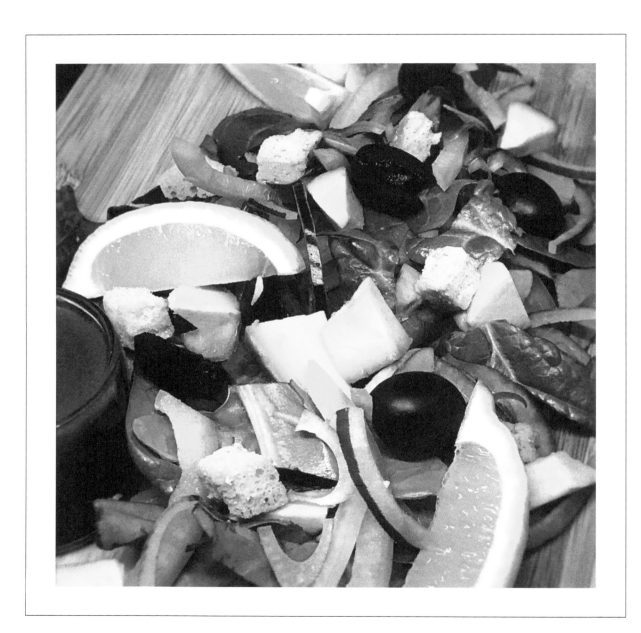

Spinach, avocado, and pepper salad

Packed full of protein and goodness, this salad is a lunch with loads of power.

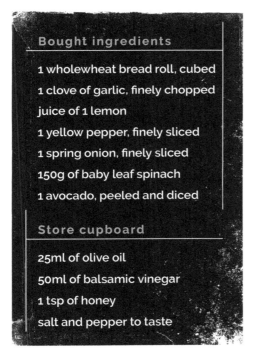

Bought ingredients

1 wholewheat bread roll, cubed

1 clove of garlic, finely chopped

juice of 1 lemon

1 yellow pepper, finely sliced

1 spring onion, finely sliced

150g of baby leaf spinach

1 avocado, peeled and diced

Store cupboard

25ml of olive oil

50ml of balsamic vinegar

1 tsp of honey

salt and pepper to taste

Putting it together

★ Preheat oven to 180 degrees Celsius.

★ Toss the bread cubes into half the olive oil and stir until they're evenly coated. Lightly season with salt and pepper and place on a lined baking tray. Bake until lightly toasted, turning once halfway through. This will take about ten minutes.

★ In a small bowl, combine the garlic, lemon juice, remaining olive oil, balsamic vinegar, and honey and mix well.

★ In a salad bowl, toss the pepper, onion, spinach, avocado, and toasted bread cubes, then pour over the dressing until everything is well coated.

Tricks and tips

This salad is delicious with grilled chicken breast (a good evening meal). Coat the chicken with olive oil and lemon juice, season to taste, and place under grill for fifteen to twenty minutes (until cooked through). You can do while toasting the bread cubes. Once cooked, slice up the chicken breast and mix into your salad.

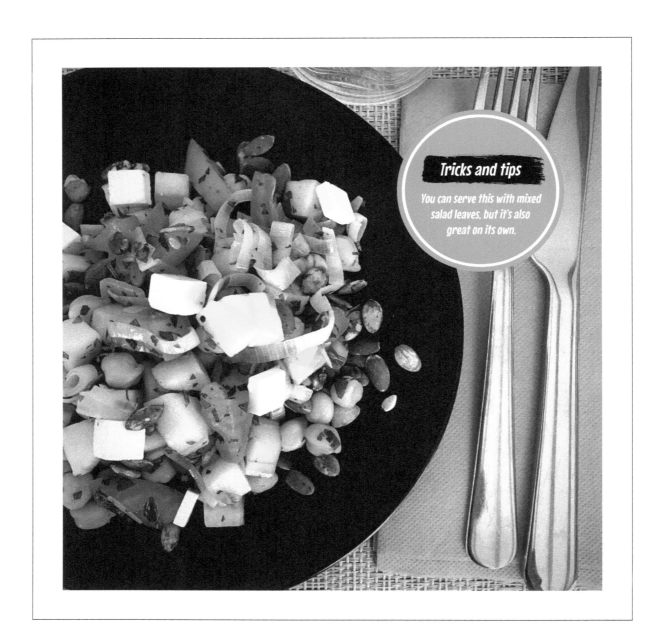

Tricks and tips

You can serve this with mixed salad leaves, but it's also great on its own.

Tomato and chickpea salad

Light and refreshing, this salad is extremely easy to prepare.

Bought ingredients	Store cupboard
2 large tomatoes, diced	25ml of olive oil
1 cucumber, peeled and diced	25ml of red wine vinegar
4 spring onions, finely sliced	1 tsp of dried oregano
1 tin of chickpeas, drained and rinsed	1 tsp of honey
50g of toasted pumpkin seeds	1 tsp of wholegrain mustard
100g of feta cheese	½ tsp of dried chilli flakes
1 tbsp of fresh parsley, finely chopped	salt and pepper to taste
juice of 1 lemon	
1 clove of garlic, finely chopped	

Putting it together

★ In a large bowl, mix the tomatoes, cucumber, onions, chickpeas, pumpkin seeds, feta cheese, and parsley.

★ Whisk the olive oil, vinegar, dried oregano and chilli flakes, honey, mustard, lemon juice, and garlic.

★ Pour dressing over salad, toss, cover, and place in the fridge to 'stand' for about an hour.

★ Season to taste.

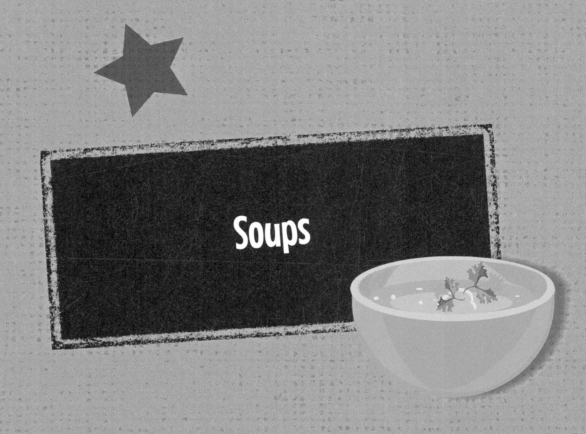

Soups

Carrot and coriander soup

A timeless classic, this soup has a slightly peppery hint.

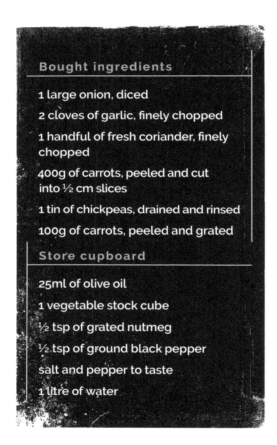

Bought ingredients

1 large onion, diced

2 cloves of garlic, finely chopped

1 handful of fresh coriander, finely chopped

400g of carrots, peeled and cut into ½ cm slices

1 tin of chickpeas, drained and rinsed

100g of carrots, peeled and grated

Store cupboard

25ml of olive oil

1 vegetable stock cube

½ tsp of grated nutmeg

½ tsp of ground black pepper

salt and pepper to taste

1 litre of water

Putting it together

★ Add the olive oil, onion, garlic, half the chopped coriander, stock cube, nutmeg, and pepper to a large saucepan and cook on low heat for about ten minutes (don't let the ingredients brown). You want the onions to soak up the spices — cooking on a low heat allows the natural juices to cook them from the inside out.

★ Add the sliced carrots and water, cover, bring to a boil, then reduce the heat and let simmer for fifteen minutes (until the carrots are tender).

★ Add the chickpeas and let simmer for five minutes, stirring gently every now and then.

★ Remove from heat and blend until smooth, then return to the saucepan and stir through the grated carrots and remaining coriander. Season to taste and serve.

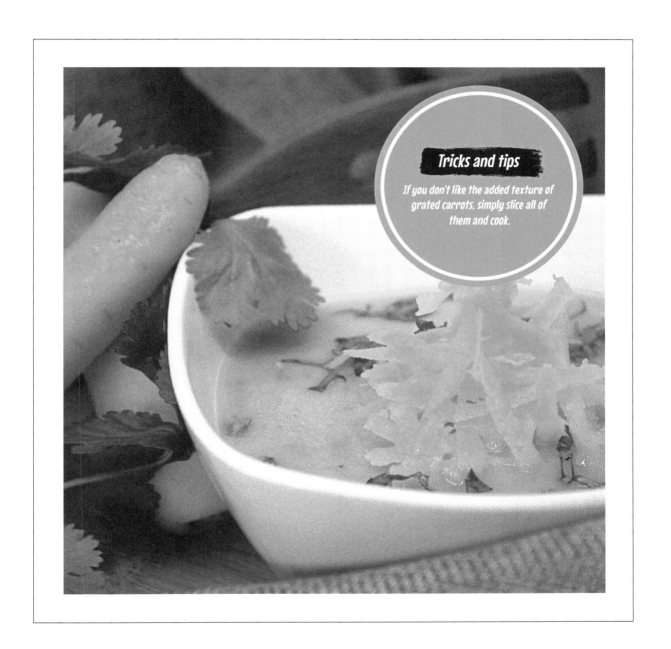

Tricks and tips

If you don't like the added texture of grated carrots, simply slice all of them and cook.

Carrot and red pepper soup

Bright, colourful, tasty!

Bought ingredients	Store cupboard
1 onion, finely diced	25ml of olive oil
1 handful of fresh parsley, finely chopped	½ tsp of salt
4 large carrots, peeled and cut into ½ cm slices	1 vegetable stock cube
1 large red pepper, diced	1 tsp of ground cumin
1 tin of chopped tomatoes	1 tsp of turmeric
1 large courgette, diced	1 tsp of ground paprika
juice and zest of 1 lemon	1 large bay leaf
	salt and pepper to taste
	1 to 2 litres of water

Putting it together

★ Heat olive oil slightly and add onion, parsley, salt, stock cube, and spices (including bay leaf). Stir until well mixed.

★ Add half a cup of water and keep stirring until the onions are soft.

★ Toss in carrots and red pepper and mix until well coated.

★ Blend the tin of chopped tomatoes with one litre of water until smooth and add to the mixture.

★ Stir until everything is well coated, add the remaining water, and boil for fifteen to twenty minutes.

★ Add courgette and cook for a further ten minutes.

★ Season to taste and stir in lemon juice and zest just before serving.

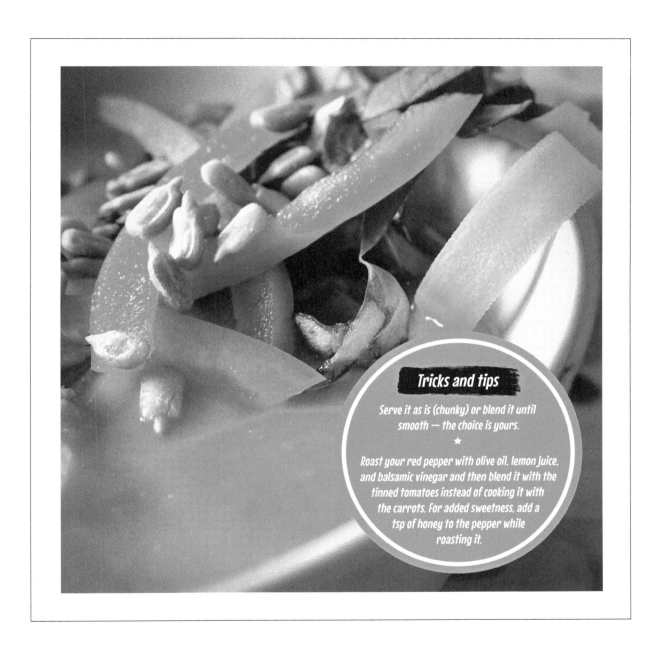

Tricks and tips

Serve it as is (chunky) or blend it until smooth — the choice is yours.

★

Roast your red pepper with olive oil, lemon juice, and balsamic vinegar and then blend it with the tinned tomatoes instead of cooking it with the carrots. For added sweetness, add a tsp of honey to the pepper while roasting it.

Cauli-broc mustard soup

There's nothing better than a rich, creamy soup, and cauliflower and mustard taste great together.

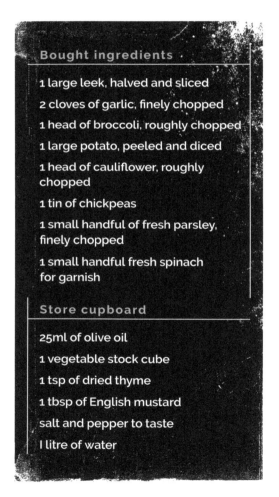

Bought ingredients

1 large leek, halved and sliced

2 cloves of garlic, finely chopped

1 head of broccoli, roughly chopped

1 large potato, peeled and diced

1 head of cauliflower, roughly chopped

1 tin of chickpeas

1 small handful of fresh parsley, finely chopped

1 small handful fresh spinach for garnish

Store cupboard

25ml of olive oil

1 vegetable stock cube

1 tsp of dried thyme

1 tbsp of English mustard

salt and pepper to taste

I litre of water

Putting it together

★ Heat the olive oil in a large saucepan, then add the leek, garlic, stock cube, and thyme and cook until the stock cube has dissolved and the leek is nice and soft.

★ Add the broccoli, potato, cauliflower, and water. Bring to the boil while stirring.

★ Simmer gently for twenty to twenty-five minutes, or until the vegetables have softened.

★ Remove from heat and, using a hand blender, mix until the soup is nice and smooth.

★ In a blender, blend the chickpeas until they're smooth and creamy. If the mixture is too thick, add a little water. We normally blend ours with the brine as well.

★ Add the creamy chickpea mixture to your soup, along with the chopped parsley and mustard, and let simmer for five minutes.

★ Season to taste and garnish with fresh parsley or finely chopped spinach.

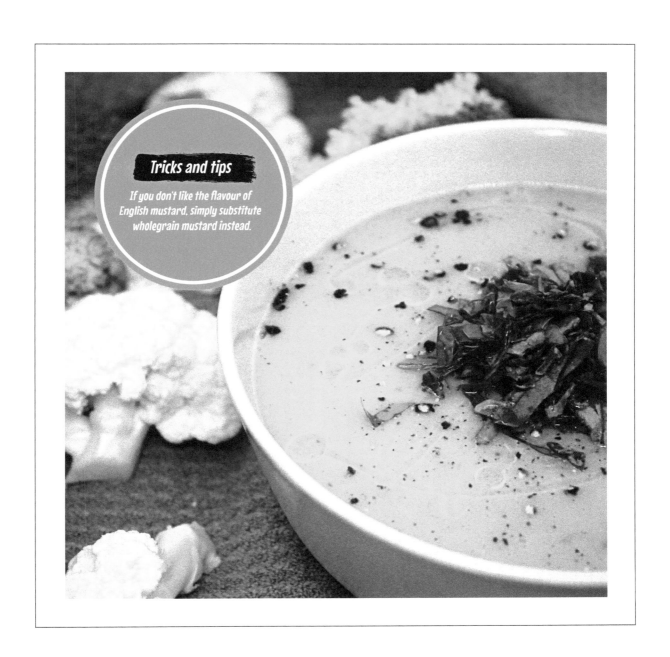

Tricks and tips

If you don't like the flavour of English mustard, simply substitute wholegrain mustard instead.

Chilli butternut squash and ginger soup

Creamy and zingy — a great soup for a chilly day.

Bought ingredients	Store cupboard
1 large butternut squash, peeled and diced	1 tbsp of butter
1 onion, diced	1 vegetable stock cube
2 cloves of garlic, finely diced	salt and pepper to taste
1" of ginger, peeled and finely chopped	750ml of water
1 small red chilli, finely chopped	
1 tin of coconut milk	
fresh coriander, roughly chopped	

Putting it together

★ Lightly heat the butter in a pan, add the butternut squash, onion, garlic, and stock cube, and stir well. Cook gently for four or five minutes.

★ Add the ginger and chilli and cook for a further five minutes.

★ Pour in the water and bring to a rapid boil, then turn down the heat slightly and simmer for about fifteen minutes, or until the squash is soft.

★ Once the squash is soft, blend until the mixture has a fine, creamy consistency.

★ Return to heat and mix in the coconut milk. Let simmer for five minutes.

★ Season to taste and garnish with fresh coriander.

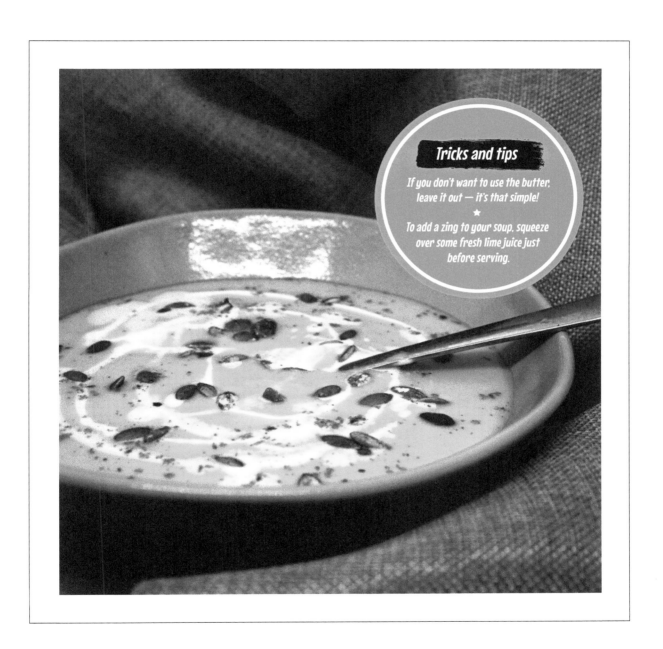

Tricks and tips

If you don't want to use the butter, leave it out — it's that simple!

★

To add a zing to your soup, squeeze over some fresh lime juice just before serving.

Chilli chickpea and lemon soup

The cumin's spicy aroma and the chillies' heat definitely make this soup a warming one.

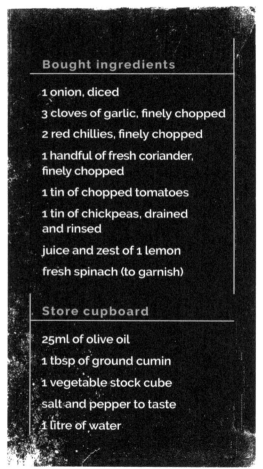

Bought ingredients

1 onion, diced

3 cloves of garlic, finely chopped

2 red chillies, finely chopped

1 handful of fresh coriander, finely chopped

1 tin of chopped tomatoes

1 tin of chickpeas, drained and rinsed

juice and zest of 1 lemon

fresh spinach (to garnish)

Store cupboard

25ml of olive oil

1 tbsp of ground cumin

1 vegetable stock cube

salt and pepper to taste

1 litre of water

Putting it together

★ Lightly heat the olive oil in a saucepan, add the onion, garlic, chillies, half the coriander, cumin and stock cube, and gently cook for five to ten minutes (until the stock cube is dissolved and the onion is soft). Stir regularly to ensure that it doesn't stick or brown.

★ Add the tinned tomatoes and cook gently for about ten minutes (until the mixture has thickened). Again, stir regularly to ensure that it doesn't stick to the pan and burn.

★ Pour in the chickpeas and water, bring to the boil, and then reduce the heat and simmer for a further fifteen minutes.

★ Remove the soup from the heat and blend half the mixture in a blender until nice and smooth.

★ Return the blended soup to the saucepan, add the lemon juice and zest and the remaining coriander, and simmer for five minutes.

★ Season to taste and garnish with freshly chopped spinach.

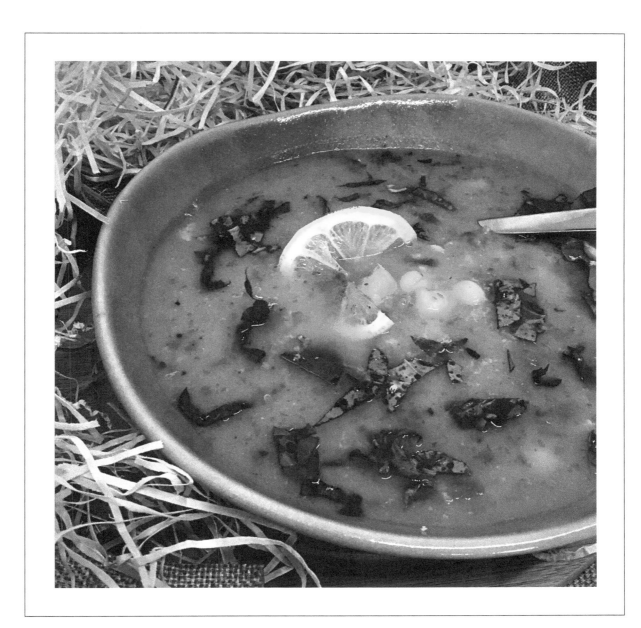

Courgette, carrot, and sweet potato soup

There are times when you might be put on the spot and need to come up with a meal based on what people can and cannot eat (i.e., allergies, food preferences). We weren't too sure about this recipe at first, but it came out really tasty.

Bought ingredients	Store cupboard
1 onion, diced	25ml of olive oil
2 cloves of garlic, finely diced	1 vegetable stock cube
450g of carrots, peeled and sliced into ½ cm slices	1 tbsp of smoked paprika
1 sweet potato, peeled and diced	salt and pepper to taste
1 handful of fresh parsley, finely chopped	chilli flakes (to garnish)
2 large courgettes, diced	1 litre of water
juice of 1 lemon	
spinach, finely chopped (to garnish)	
toasted pumpkin seeds (to garnish)	

Putting it together

★ Gently heat the olive oil in a large saucepan with the onion, garlic, vegetable stock cube, and paprika for two to three minutes, until the onions have softened and the stock cube has dissolved.

★ Add the carrots, sweet potato, parsley, and water. Bring to the boil then simmer for fifteen to twenty minutes, until the vegetables are tender.

★ Add the courgette and let simmer for a further ten minutes (until tender).

★ Remove the saucepan from the heat, pour the soup into a blender, and blend until it's creamy and smooth.

★ Return to the heat, add the lemon juice, and let simmer for five minutes.

★ Season to taste and garnish with a pinch of fresh spinach, some pumpkin seeds, and a sprinkle of chilli flakes.

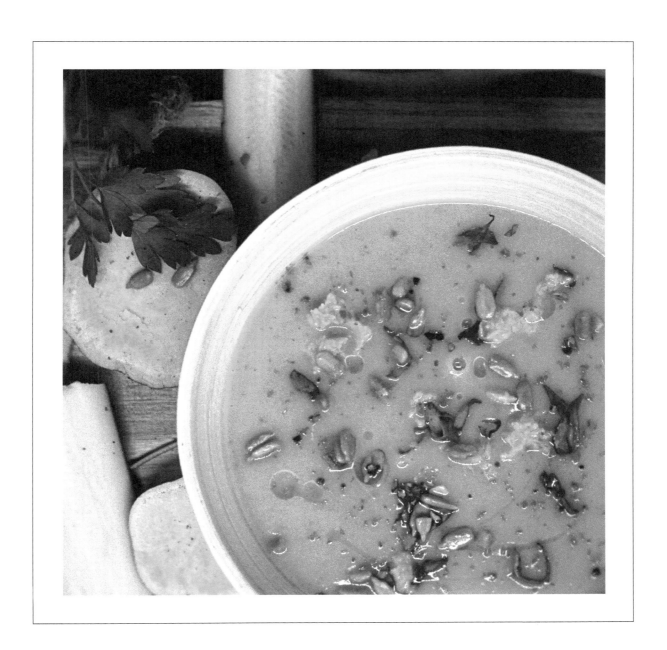

Courgette, pea, and cannellini bean soup

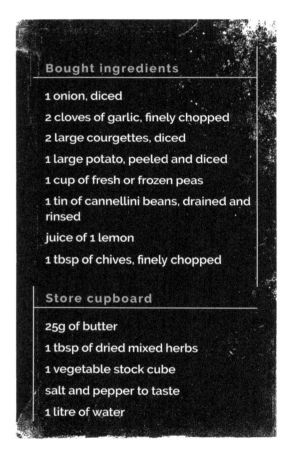

Bought ingredients

1 onion, diced

2 cloves of garlic, finely chopped

2 large courgettes, diced

1 large potato, peeled and diced

1 cup of fresh or frozen peas

1 tin of cannellini beans, drained and rinsed

juice of 1 lemon

1 tbsp of chives, finely chopped

Store cupboard

25g of butter

1 tbsp of dried mixed herbs

1 vegetable stock cube

salt and pepper to taste

1 litre of water

Putting it together

★ In a large saucepan, melt the butter, add the onion, garlic, courgettes, mixed herbs, and stock cube, and cook gently for five to six minutes (until the onions are golden brown and the stock cube has dissolved).

★ Add the potato and half the water and simmer for ten to fifteen minutes (until the potatoes are slightly cooked).

★ Add the peas, cannellini beans, and lemon juice along with the remaining water and bring to the boil. Let simmer for a further ten minutes.

★ Remove from heat and blend the soup until smooth.

★ Return to the saucepan, add the chives, and let simmer for five minutes.

★ Season to taste.

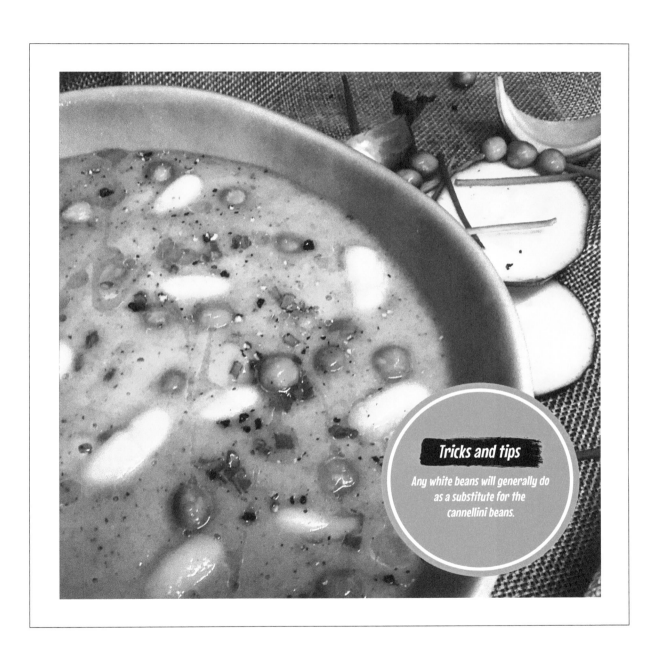

Tricks and tips

Any white beans will generally do as a substitute for the cannellini beans.

Courgette, pea, and mint soup

Refreshingly tasty!

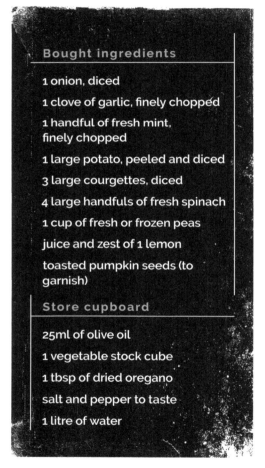

Bought ingredients

1 onion, diced

1 clove of garlic, finely chopped

1 handful of fresh mint, finely chopped

1 large potato, peeled and diced

3 large courgettes, diced

4 large handfuls of fresh spinach

1 cup of fresh or frozen peas

juice and zest of 1 lemon

toasted pumpkin seeds (to garnish)

Store cupboard

25ml of olive oil

1 vegetable stock cube

1 tbsp of dried oregano

salt and pepper to taste

1 litre of water

Putting it together

★ Lightly heat the oil in a large saucepan, add the onion, garlic, mint, stock cube, and dried oregano, and cook for five minutes until the stock cube is dissolved and the onion is soft.

★ Add the potato and cover and cook for five to ten minutes, stirring occasionally to prevent sticking and to stop the potatoes from browning. If the mixture is too dry, add a splash of water.

★ Add the courgettes and mix until everything is nicely coated.

★ Pour in the water, bring to the boil, then cover and simmer for about fifteen minutes.

★ Add the spinach, peas, and lemon juice and zest and cook for a further five minutes.

★ Remove from heat and blend until the soup is smooth and creamy. Season to taste.

★ Reheat gently for about three minutes and then garnish with finely sliced spinach, a drizzle of lemon juice and olive oil, and some toasted pumpkin seeds for crunch.

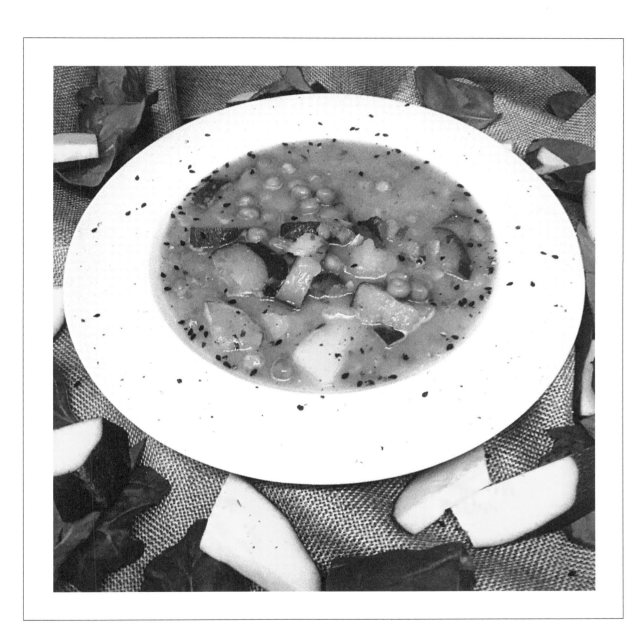

D-Toxd vegetable soup

There's nothing better than a steaming bowl of vegetable soup on a cold winter's evening. Make sure you add a big dose of love while preparing this recipe — it goes a long way in a soup like this, because it is so homely and chunky and 'just like Grandma used to make'."

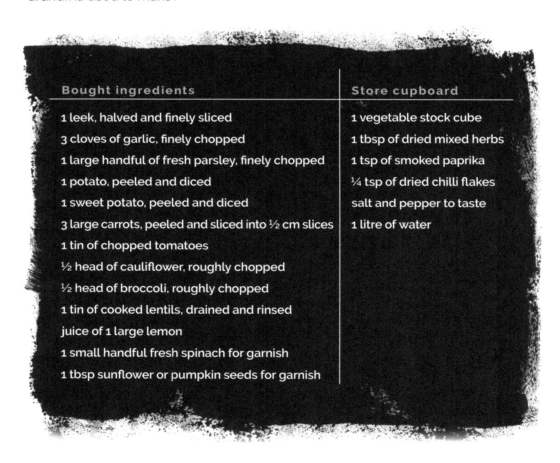

Bought ingredients	Store cupboard
1 leek, halved and finely sliced	1 vegetable stock cube
3 cloves of garlic, finely chopped	1 tbsp of dried mixed herbs
1 large handful of fresh parsley, finely chopped	1 tsp of smoked paprika
1 potato, peeled and diced	¼ tsp of dried chilli flakes
1 sweet potato, peeled and diced	salt and pepper to taste
3 large carrots, peeled and sliced into ½ cm slices	1 litre of water
1 tin of chopped tomatoes	
½ head of cauliflower, roughly chopped	
½ head of broccoli, roughly chopped	
1 tin of cooked lentils, drained and rinsed	
juice of 1 large lemon	
1 small handful fresh spinach for garnish	
1 tbsp sunflower or pumpkin seeds for garnish	

Putting it together

* In a large saucepan, lightly steam-fry (using a small amount of water) the stock cube, mixed herbs, paprika, chilli flakes, leek, garlic, and parsley until the stock cube is dissolved and the leeks are soft.

* Throw in the potatoes and carrots and stir until well coated with leek mixture.

* Pour in the tinned tomatoes and mix well.

* Add the water and bring to the boil, then reduce heat and simmer for about ten to fifteen minutes (or until the vegetables are cooked). You want the vegetables to be al dente.

* Add the cauliflower and cook slightly.

* Throw in the broccoli and let simmer gently for three or four minutes.

* Add the lentils and lemon juice and simmer for a few minutes so that the lentils are warmed through.

* Season to taste.

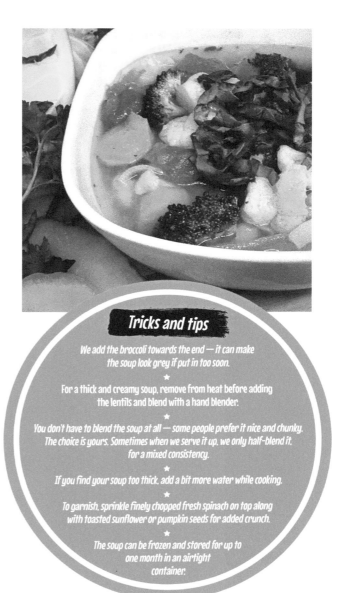

Tricks and tips

We add the broccoli towards the end — it can make the soup look grey if put in too soon.

★

For a thick and creamy soup, remove from heat before adding the lentils and blend with a hand blender.

★

You don't have to blend the soup at all — some people prefer it nice and chunky. The choice is yours. Sometimes when we serve it up, we only half-blend it for a mixed consistency.

★

If you find your soup too thick, add a bit more water while cooking.

★

To garnish, sprinkle finely chopped fresh spinach on top along with toasted sunflower or pumpkin seeds for added crunch.

★

The soup can be frozen and stored for up to one month in an airtight container.

Detox superfood green vegetable soup

This soup is ideal if you want to give your body a good cleanse; it's packed full of green goodness — so much so that Popeye eats it in cold weather.

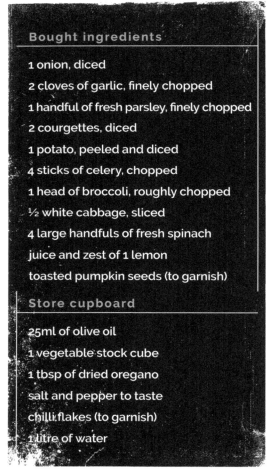

Bought ingredients

1 onion, diced

2 cloves of garlic, finely chopped

1 handful of fresh parsley, finely chopped

2 courgettes, diced

1 potato, peeled and diced

4 sticks of celery, chopped

1 head of broccoli, roughly chopped

½ white cabbage, sliced

4 large handfuls of fresh spinach

juice and zest of 1 lemon

toasted pumpkin seeds (to garnish)

Store cupboard

25ml of olive oil

1 vegetable stock cube

1 tbsp of dried oregano

salt and pepper to taste

chilli flakes (to garnish)

1 litre of water

Putting it together

★ In a large saucepan, lightly heat the olive oil, then gently fry the onion, garlic, half the chopped parsley, vegetable stock cube, and oregano until the onions are soft and tender and the stock cube has dissolved.

★ Add the courgettes, potato, and celery with a small amount of water (about 50ml) and gently stir, coating the vegetables well with the onion mixture.

★ Add the broccoli, cabbage, lemon zest, and half the spinach, mix everything, then pour in the remaining water and bring to the boil.

★ Reduce the heat and simmer for fifteen to twenty minutes.

★ Remove the saucepan from the heat, add the soup to a blender, and blend until it's creamy and smooth.

★ Return to the heat, add the lemon juice and remaining parsley and spinach, and let simmer for five minutes.

★ Season to taste and garnish with a pinch of fresh spinach, some pumpkin seeds, and a sprinkle of chilli flakes.

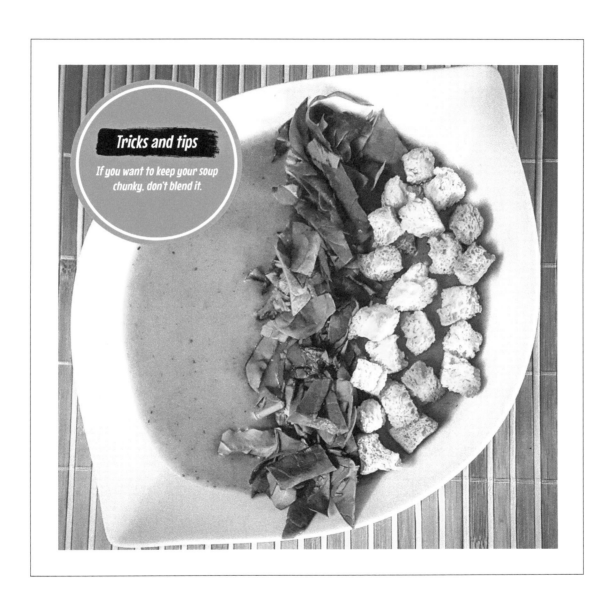

Tricks and tips

If you want to keep your soup chunky, don't blend it.

Leek, asparagus, and baby potato soup

A delicious soup for a cold evening.

Bought ingredients	Store cupboard
1 leek, halved and finely sliced (we use only the white part)	1 tbsp of butter
1 clove of garlic, finely chopped	1 tbsp of dried mixed herbs
300g of baby potatoes, diced	½ tsp of dried tarragon
2 bunches of asparagus, tips removed and stalks cut into 1" lengths	1 vegetable stock cube
1 tin of chickpeas, drained and rinsed	salt and pepper to taste
squeeze of lemon juice	1 litre water
1 small handful of fresh parsley, finely chopped	

Putting it together

★ In a large saucepan, melt the butter and add the leek, garlic, mixed herbs, tarragon, and stock cube and cook until the stock cube is melted and the leeks are soft.

★ Add the potatoes and water, bring to the boil while stirring gently, then reduce heat and let simmer for fifteen minutes (until the potatoes are almost cooked through).

★ Stir in the asparagus stalks and chickpeas and let simmer for a further ten minutes (until the asparagus is cooked through and the chickpeas start to break down).

★ While the soup is cooking, either steam or boil the asparagus tips and set aside to use as a flavour-filled garnish. Season them with a squeeze of lemon juice and some black pepper.

★ Remove half the soup and blend in a blender until it's smooth and creamy.

★ Return the blended soup to the saucepan, add the chopped parsley, and season to taste. Let simmer for three or four minutes before serving.

★ Garnish with asparagus tips and chopped parsley.

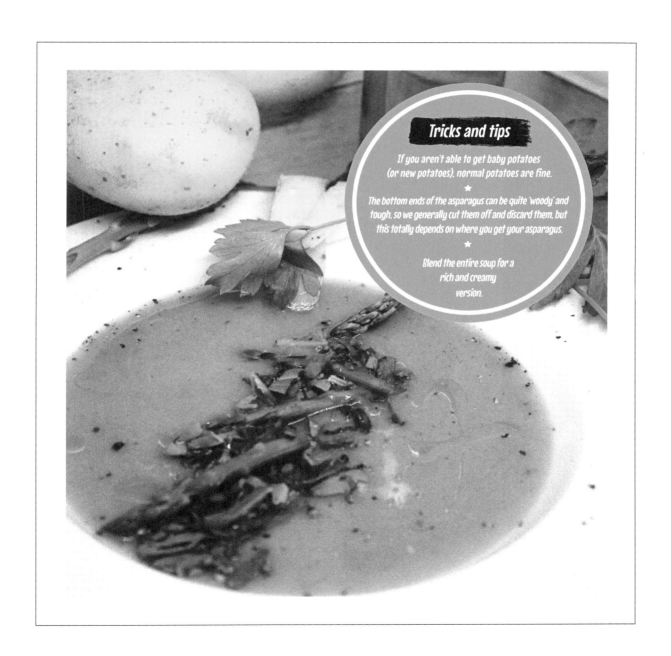

Tricks and tips

If you aren't able to get baby potatoes (or new potatoes), normal potatoes are fine.

★

The bottom ends of the asparagus can be quite 'woody' and tough, so we generally cut them off and discard them, but this totally depends on where you get your asparagus.

★

Blend the entire soup for a rich and creamy version.

Potato, asparagus, pea, and mint soup

The fresh flavours of this soup, combined with its glowing colour, make it a truly enticing dish.

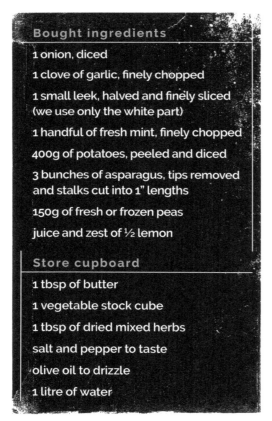

Bought ingredients

1 onion, diced

1 clove of garlic, finely chopped

1 small leek, halved and finely sliced (we use only the white part)

1 handful of fresh mint, finely chopped

400g of potatoes, peeled and diced

3 bunches of asparagus, tips removed and stalks cut into 1" lengths

150g of fresh or frozen peas

juice and zest of ½ lemon

Store cupboard

1 tbsp of butter

1 vegetable stock cube

1 tbsp of dried mixed herbs

salt and pepper to taste

olive oil to drizzle

1 litre of water

Putting it together

★ Gently heat the butter in a large saucepan.

★ Add the onion, garlic, and leek, half the mint, the stock cube, and the mixed herbs and cook for five minutes (until the stock cube is dissolved and the leeks and onion are soft).

★ Add the potatoes, cover, and cook for five to ten minutes, stirring occasionally to prevent sticking and to stop the potatoes from browning. If the mixture is too dry, add a splash of water — you want the potatoes to absorb the flavours.

★ Pour in the water and chopped asparagus, bring to the boil, then cover and simmer for about five minutes (until the asparagus is tender).

★ Add the remaining mint, peas and juice and zest of half a lemon and cook for a further five minutes.

★ While the soup is cooking, either steam or boil the asparagus tips and set aside for garnish. Season with a squeeze of lemon juice and some black pepper.

★ Remove the soup from the heat and blend until smooth and creamy.

★ Reheat gently for about three minutes and then garnish with the asparagus tips and a drizzle of lemon juice and olive oil.

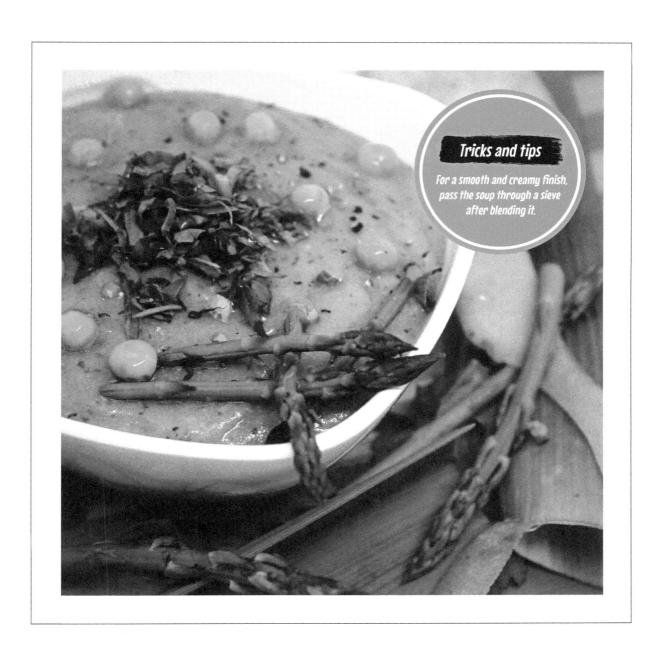

Tricks and tips

For a smooth and creamy finish, pass the soup through a sieve after blending it.

Roast red pepper and tomato soup

Roasting always brings out the fresh flavours in vegetables. Take time with the roasting and this soup will be even tastier.

Bought ingredients	Store cupboard
1 kg of fresh tomatoes, quartered	25ml of olive oil
2 large red peppers, diced	50ml of balsamic vinegar
2 red onions, roughly chopped	2 tbsp of honey
4 cloves of garlic, roughly chopped	1 tsp of smoked paprika
1 handful of fresh parsley, roughly chopped	1 tsp of ground pimento
1 tbsp of fresh rosemary, roughly chopped	1 tsp of ground black pepper
juice of 2 lemons	1 tsp of sea salt
zest of 1 lemon	½ tsp of dried chilli flakes
fresh basil (to garnish)	125ml of water

Putting it together

★ Preheat oven to 180 degrees Celsius — cooking slowly on a low temperature brings all the flavours together.

★ On a roasting tray, combine all the ingredients (except the water) and mix well so that everything is nicely blended.

★ Place in the middle of the oven and cook for about one and a half hours, checking it every twenty minutes or so and giving it a stir.

★ Once the vegetables are cooked, place everything in a blender and blend until smooth. If the tomatoes are a little dry and the 'sauce' is a little sticky, this means the vegetables are cooked. Don't cook so long that the vegetables dry out.

★ Place in a saucepan with the water and lightly simmer for a few minutes.

★ Season to taste and served garnished with some fresh basil.

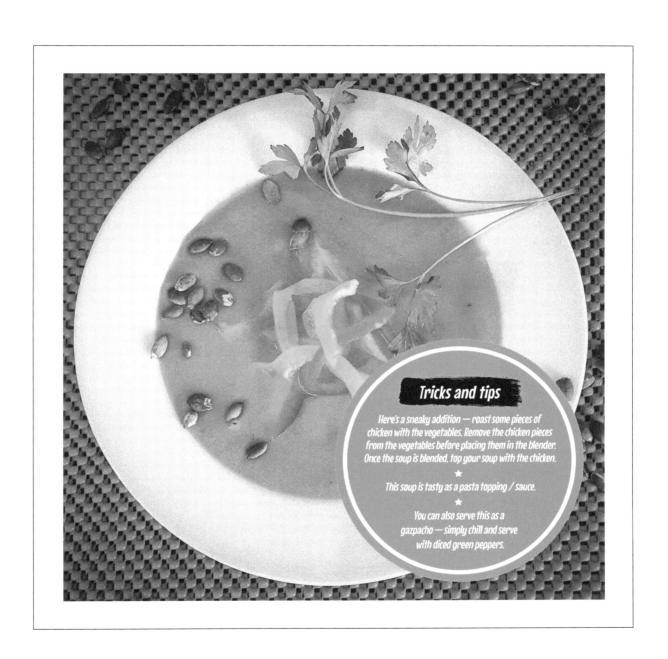

Tricks and tips

Here's a sneaky addition — roast some pieces of chicken with the vegetables. Remove the chicken pieces from the vegetables before placing them in the blender. Once the soup is blended, top your soup with the chicken.

★

This soup is tasty as a pasta topping / sauce.

★

You can also serve this as a gazpacho — simply chill and serve with diced green peppers.

Roast tomato and basil soup

The combination of herbs and the sweetness and tanginess of the honey, lemon juice, and balsamic vinegar make this a warming soup bursting with colour and taste.

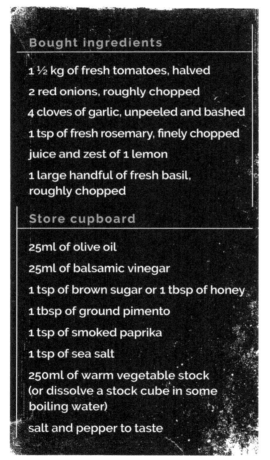

Bought ingredients

1 ½ kg of fresh tomatoes, halved

2 red onions, roughly chopped

4 cloves of garlic, unpeeled and bashed

1 tsp of fresh rosemary, finely chopped

juice and zest of 1 lemon

1 large handful of fresh basil, roughly chopped

Store cupboard

25ml of olive oil

25ml of balsamic vinegar

1 tsp of brown sugar or 1 tbsp of honey

1 tbsp of ground pimento

1 tsp of smoked paprika

1 tsp of sea salt

250ml of warm vegetable stock (or dissolve a stock cube in some boiling water)

salt and pepper to taste

Putting it together

★ Preheat oven to 200 degrees Celsius.

★ To bash your garlic, turn your knife on its side and press down on the clove.

★ Place the tomatoes, onions, garlic, rosemary, lemon zest, and half the basil into a roasting tray, then pour over the olive oil, balsamic vinegar, sugar or honey, spices, and sea salt. Toss until everything is nicely coated.

★ Place in oven and roast for forty-five minutes to an hour, checking it every now and then and giving it a slight stir when needed. The tomatoes and onions will be soft when it's ready.

★ Remove from the oven, peel the roasted garlic and place in a blender with the roasted vegetables, lemon juice, and vegetable stock and blend until smooth.

★ Place in a saucepan, reheat, and simmer for five minutes.

★ Season to taste and garnish with chopped basil and lemon zest.

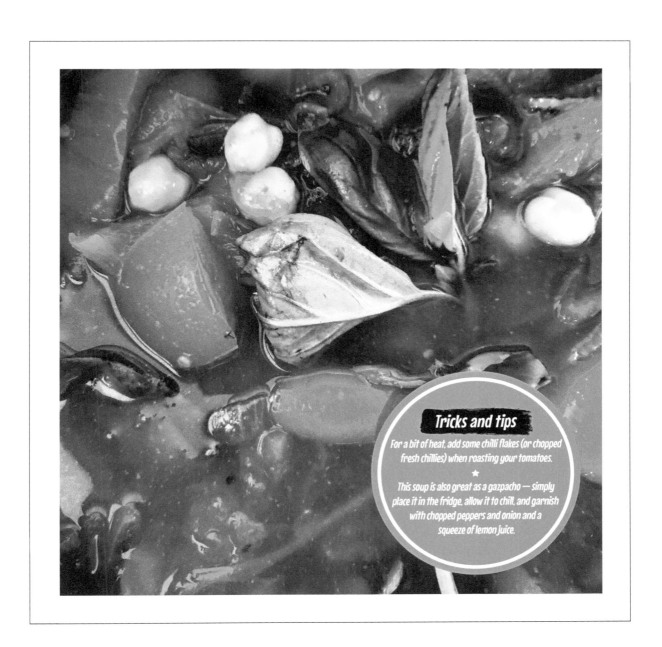

Tricks and tips

For a bit of heat, add some chilli flakes (or chopped fresh chillies) when roasting your tomatoes.

★

This soup is also great as a gazpacho — simply place it in the fridge, allow it to chill, and garnish with chopped peppers and onion and a squeeze of lemon juice.

Spicy sweet potato soup

Sweet and chilli is always a great combination. Add some zesty ginger and lime to the duo and you have a taste sensation.

Bought ingredients	Store cupboard
1 onion, diced	25ml of olive oil
1 clove of garlic, finely chopped	1 vegetable stock cube
2 red chillies, finely chopped	2 tsp of ground ginger
1 handful of fresh coriander, finely chopped	½ tsp of cayenne pepper
2 large sweet potatoes, peeled and diced	¼ tsp of ground cumin
	¼ tsp of ground cinnamon
1 large potato, peeled and diced	2 tbsp of honey
1 large red pepper, diced	salt and pepper to taste
juice of 2 limes	black sesame seeds (to garnish; optional)
	1 litre of water

Putting it together

★ In a large saucepan, gently fry the olive oil, onion, garlic, chillies, half the coriander, the stock cube, all the spices, and the honey (until the onions are soft and the stock cube is dissolved).

★ Add the potatoes and red pepper and stir for two to three minutes (until everything is coated with the mixture and the red peppers have started to soften).

★ Pour in the water and bring to the boil, then reduce the heat, cover, and let simmer for fifteen to twenty minutes (until the potatoes are cooked).

★ Remove from heat and blend until smooth.

★ Return to the stove, add the remaining coriander and the lime juice, and let simmer gently for another five minutes, stirring well to mix through the herbs.

★ Season to taste and garnish with chopped coriander, a squeeze of lime juice, and a sprinkle of black sesame seeds.

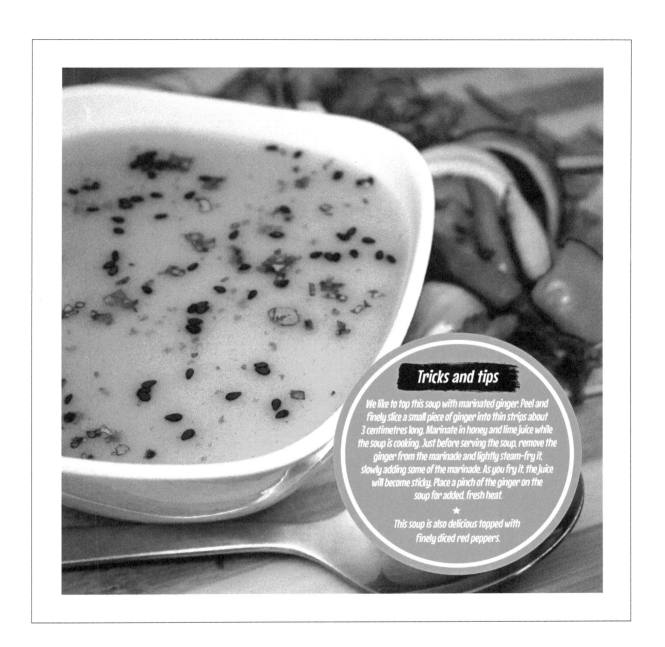

Tricks and tips

We like to top this soup with marinated ginger. Peel and finely slice a small piece of ginger into thin strips about 3 centimetres long. Marinate in honey and lime juice while the soup is cooking. Just before serving the soup, remove the ginger from the marinade and lightly steam-fry it, slowly adding some of the marinade. As you fry it, the juice will become sticky. Place a pinch of the ginger on the soup for added, fresh heat.

★

This soup is also delicious topped with finely diced red peppers.

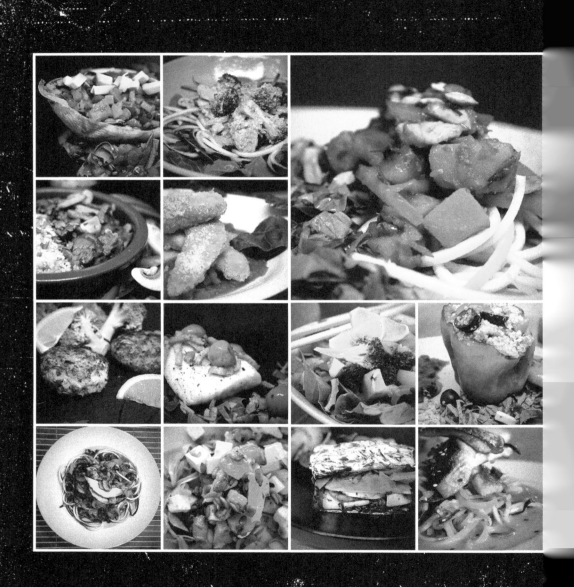

ROCKET FUEL:
THE MAIN MEALS

Whether you're eating on your own, with friends, or with family members, you likely don't have hours and hours (and sometimes hours) to prepare meals. You probably want something that looks great, tastes amazing, and is good for you but, above all else, is easy to put together.

As we mentioned at the start of the book, we're *not* chefs! We haven't trained in cooking. It's something that, over time, we've truly embraced and learned to enjoy. We have to deliver meals to our guests in a finite amount of time while still doing everything else necessary to keep our retreat going. For that reason, we've found ways to make sure these meals don't take ages to prepare.

Some of the meals will take a little more effort than others, but with some practice, you'll be cooking them like a champ in no time.

Recipes in this section

MEALS

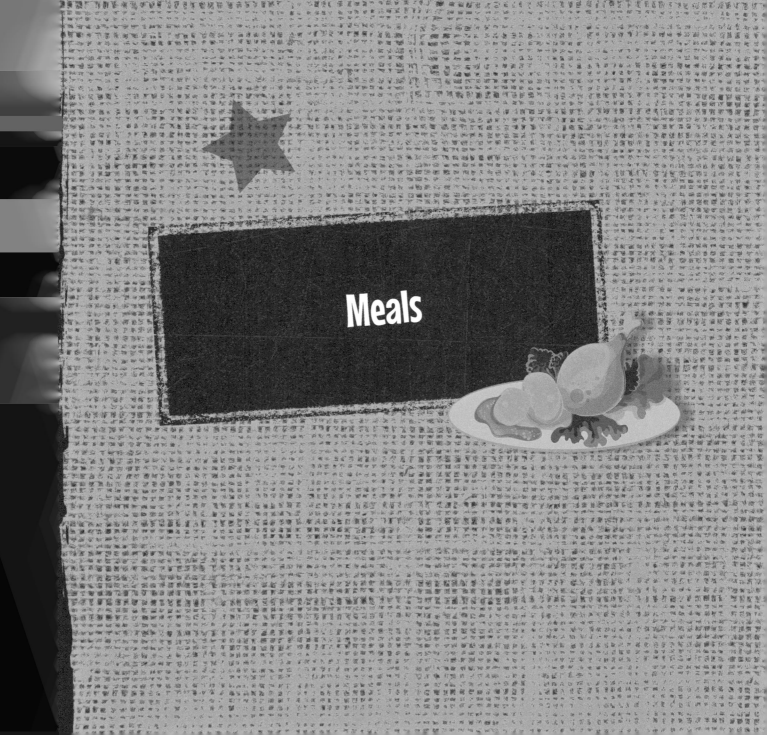

Meals

Anne's oven-baked aubergine with olive and caper sauce

This dish was inspired by a friend who came out to the retreat and prepared it for us during her stay.

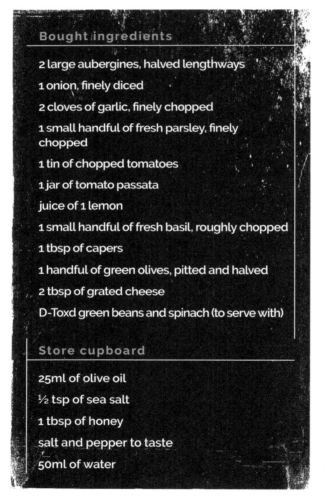

Bought ingredients

2 large aubergines, halved lengthways

1 onion, finely diced

2 cloves of garlic, finely chopped

1 small handful of fresh parsley, finely chopped

1 tin of chopped tomatoes

1 jar of tomato passata

juice of 1 lemon

1 small handful of fresh basil, roughly chopped

1 tbsp of capers

1 handful of green olives, pitted and halved

2 tbsp of grated cheese

D-Toxd green beans and spinach (to serve with)

Store cupboard

25ml of olive oil

½ tsp of sea salt

1 tbsp of honey

salt and pepper to taste

50ml of water

Putting it together

★ Preheat oven to 200 degrees Celsius. For fan ovens, preheat to 180 degrees C.

★ Drizzle the aubergines with olive oil, lightly season with salt and pepper, place in an ovenproof dish, and bake for about thirty to thirty-five minutes, or until soft.

★ While the aubergines are cooking, lightly heat the olive oil in a saucepan and gently fry the onion, garlic, parsley, and salt for about five minutes (until the onions are soft and tender).

★ Add the tomatoes and honey and gently cook for another three or four minutes (until the tomatoes have reduced slightly).

★ Add the passata, lemon juice, and water, bring to the boil, then reduce heat and simmer for about ten minutes, to let the mixture thicken.

★ Mix through the capers, olives, and half the fresh basil, season

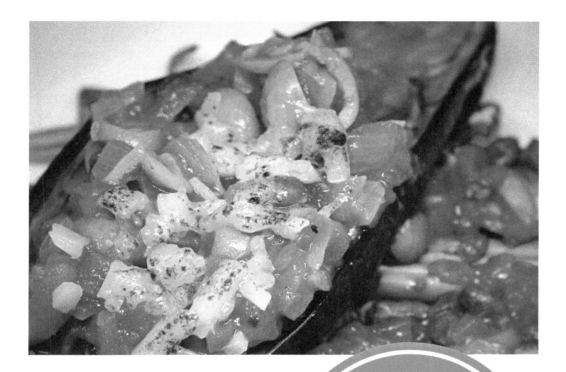

to taste, and let stand for at least ten minutes.

★ Pour two tbsp of the sauce over each of the aubergine halves, top with cheese, and return to the oven for another ten minutes so that the cheese melts and the aubergines finish cooking.

★ Remove from heat, garnish with remaining basil, and serve with D-Toxd green beans and spinach (see recipe in this section, accompanied by more of the sauce).

Tricks and tips

To give your sauce a bit more depth, add red wine during the cooking process. When it reduces, it releases flavours that complement the tomatoes and aubergines.
Add the wine with your tomatoes and honey and allow it to reduce before adding the passata and lemon juice.

★

Leftover sauce is great served with courgette spaghetti for a quick meal.

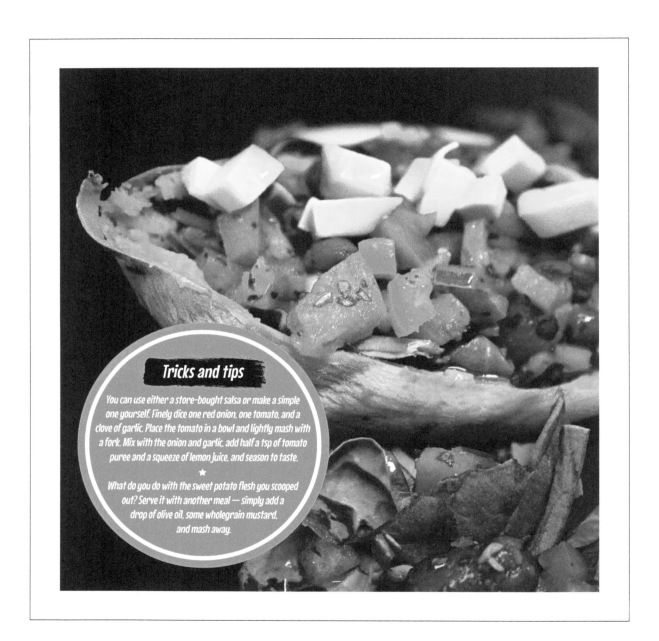

Tricks and tips

You can use either a store-bought salsa or make a simple one yourself. Finely dice one red onion, one tomato, and a clove of garlic. Place the tomato in a bowl and lightly mash with a fork. Mix with the onion and garlic, add half a tsp of tomato puree and a squeeze of lemon juice, and season to taste.

★

What do you do with the sweet potato flesh you scooped out? Serve it with another meal — simply add a drop of olive oil, some wholegrain mustard, and mash away.

Baked salsa sweet potato bowls

Everyone loves a baked potato, but how often do you have one that's tasty and refreshing and doesn't give you that 'carb crash'?

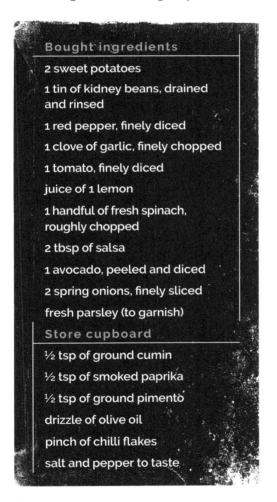

Bought ingredients

2 sweet potatoes

1 tin of kidney beans, drained and rinsed

1 red pepper, finely diced

1 clove of garlic, finely chopped

1 tomato, finely diced

juice of 1 lemon

1 handful of fresh spinach, roughly chopped

2 tbsp of salsa

1 avocado, peeled and diced

2 spring onions, finely sliced

fresh parsley (to garnish)

Store cupboard

½ tsp of ground cumin

½ tsp of smoked paprika

½ tsp of ground pimento

drizzle of olive oil

pinch of chilli flakes

salt and pepper to taste

Putting it together

★ Preheat the oven to 200 degrees Celsius.

★ Wash the sweet potatoes and stab them with a fork a few times. Bake for about an hour (until they're soft to the touch).

★ While the potatoes are baking, place the beans, pepper, spring onions, garlic, tomato, lemon juice, and spices in a bowl and mix well.

★ When the potatoes are done, slice them in half and let them cool down. Using a tbsp, scoop out some of the flesh to form a bowl (leave about 1 to 1 ½ centimetres of potato).

★ Place half a handful of fresh spinach in the scooped out sweet potatoes, followed by the vegetable mixture. Top with salsa, avocado, and spring onions.

★ Drizzle over a little oil and a pinch of chilli flakes and place under the grill for a few minutes, so that the avocado turns slightly golden.

★ Season to taste and garnish with fresh parsley.

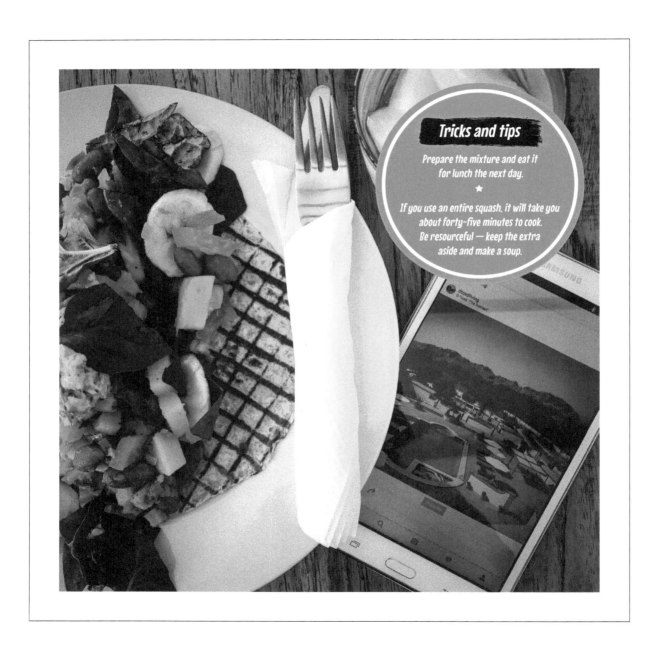

Tricks and tips

Prepare the mixture and eat it for lunch the next day.

★

If you use an entire squash, it will take you about forty-five minutes to cook. Be resourceful — keep the extra aside and make a soup.

Banana and kidney bean wraps

Great wraps for a Saturday night while watching a movie and relaxing. They're simple. They're delicious. And even better? They're like 'junk food' — but with a massive boost of nutrients and energy.

And don't be put off by the ingredients! They're surprisingly good together.

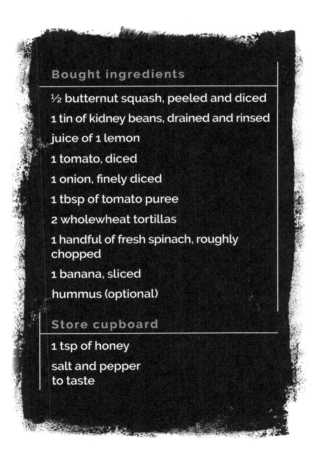

Bought ingredients

½ butternut squash, peeled and diced

1 tin of kidney beans, drained and rinsed

juice of 1 lemon

1 tomato, diced

1 onion, finely diced

1 tbsp of tomato puree

2 wholewheat tortillas

1 handful of fresh spinach, roughly chopped

1 banana, sliced

hummus (optional)

Store cupboard

1 tsp of honey

salt and pepper to taste

Putting it together

★ Preheat oven to 200 degrees Celsius and bake the squash for ten to twelve minutes (until cooked through). The smaller your cubes, the quicker they'll cook, but don't make them too small or they'll break apart (we usually cut ours into 1-centimetre cubes).

★ In a bowl, mix the kidney beans, lemon juice, tomato, onion, tomato puree, and honey until the beans are nicely coated.

★ Place the wraps in the oven and warm to your desired temperature.

★ Place the heated wraps on a flat surface and layer them up — a handful of spinach, some roasted butternut squash, kidney bean mixture, and hummus, and finally, some sliced banana.

★ Season to taste, wrap it up, and enjoy.

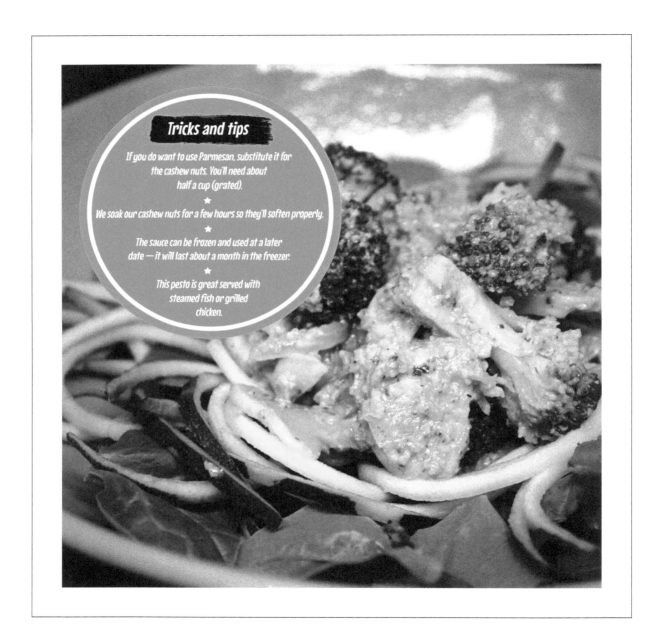

Tricks and tips

If you do want to use Parmesan, substitute it for the cashew nuts. You'll need about half a cup (grated).

★

We soak our cashew nuts for a few hours so they'll soften properly.

★

The sauce can be frozen and used at a later date — it will last about a month in the freezer.

★

This pesto is great served with steamed fish or grilled chicken.

Broccoli and cashew nut pesto sauce with mushrooms

Traditional pesto calls for Parmesan cheese. For this version, we use cashew nuts. They give the sauce a delicious, cheesy flavour, which tastes awesome with the smoked paprika.

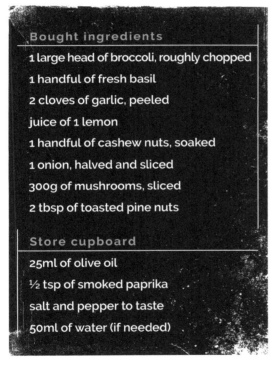

Bought ingredients

1 large head of broccoli, roughly chopped

1 handful of fresh basil

2 cloves of garlic, peeled

juice of 1 lemon

1 handful of cashew nuts, soaked

1 onion, halved and sliced

300g of mushrooms, sliced

2 tbsp of toasted pine nuts

Store cupboard

25ml of olive oil

½ tsp of smoked paprika

salt and pepper to taste

50ml of water (if needed)

Putting it together

★ Cut the broccoli into florets and steam or boil until al dente (overcooking the broccoli will make the dish soggy and grey).

★ Place half the steamed broccoli into a blender with the basil, garlic, lemon juice, cashew nuts, olive oil, and smoked paprika and blend until smooth. If the mixture seems too thick, add a little water.

★ In a large pan, lightly fry the onion slices until they're soft and slightly see-through.

★ Mix in the mushrooms and cook on a low heat for two or three minutes, then add the remaining broccoli.

★ Pour the broccoli pesto into the onions and mushrooms and mix. Warm through gently.

★ To toast the pine nuts, simply heat up a frying pan, toss them in, and shake the pan around to ensure they don't stick. After a few moments, if the pan is hot enough, they'll start to turn golden brown. You don't need any oil as pine nuts are naturally oily.

★ Serve your pesto with courgette or sweet potato spaghetti and sprinkle toasted pine nuts on top.

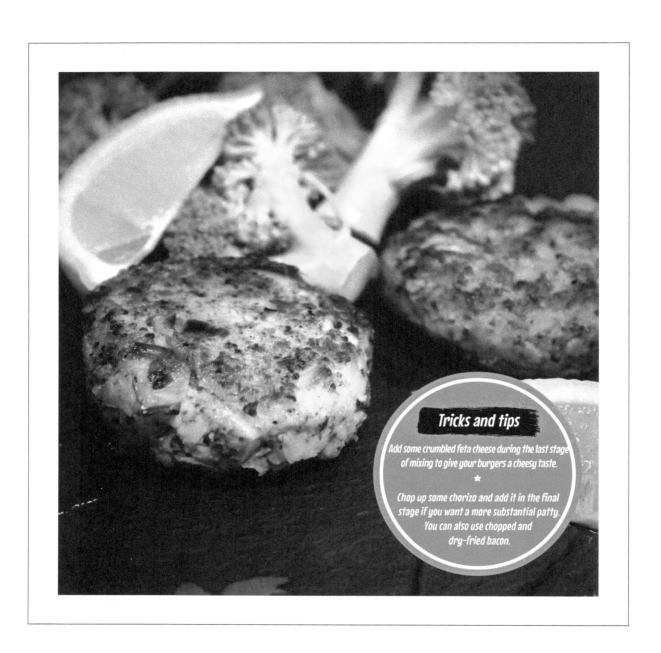

Tricks and tips

Add some crumbled feta cheese during the last stage of mixing to give your burgers a cheesy taste.

★

Chop up some chorizo and add it in the final stage if you want a more substantial patty. You can also use chopped and dry-fried bacon.

Broccoli and chickpea burgers

These are a healthy substitute for those energy-less, quick burgers we sometimes go for, and they're easy to prepare. They're also great as a quick snack — throw them in a lightly toasted pitta with some fresh green salad and a dollop of tzatziki. We've even heard that kids enjoy these burgers!

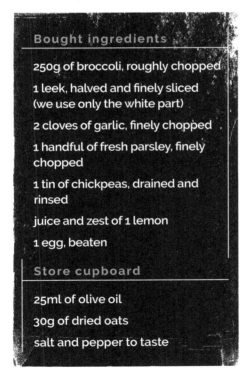

Bought ingredients

250g of broccoli, roughly chopped

1 leek, halved and finely sliced (we use only the white part)

2 cloves of garlic, finely chopped

1 handful of fresh parsley, finely chopped

1 tin of chickpeas, drained and rinsed

juice and zest of 1 lemon

1 egg, beaten

Store cupboard

25ml of olive oil

30g of dried oats

salt and pepper to taste

Putting it together

★ Steam the broccoli for three to four minutes (until it's just cooked — you don't want it too soggy or too firm).

★ Heat the oil in a frying pan with the leek and garlic and cook for three to four minutes (until softened).

★ Remove the broccoli tops (the flowery part) and set aside for use later on (to give your burgers some texture and 'meat').

★ Place the broccoli stalks, leek and garlic mixture, parsley, chickpeas, and lemon juice and zest into a food processor and blitz until it forms a rough paste — don't mix it for too long or it will turn to mush. If you don't have a food processor, put the items in a bowl and get mashing.

★ Preheat oven to 180 degrees Celsius (unless you'd rather fry the burgers).

★ Place the blended mixture into a large mixing bowl. Add the egg, oats, and broccoli tops and mix until everything is well blended. If the texture is too mushy, or there's too much liquid, add more oats to firm it up.

★ Now for the fun part! Using your hands, shape the mixture into patties and place on a lightly oiled baking tray.

★ Bake for ten to twelve minutes (until crisp), or you can lightly fry them in a small amount of olive oil for three to four minutes on each side.

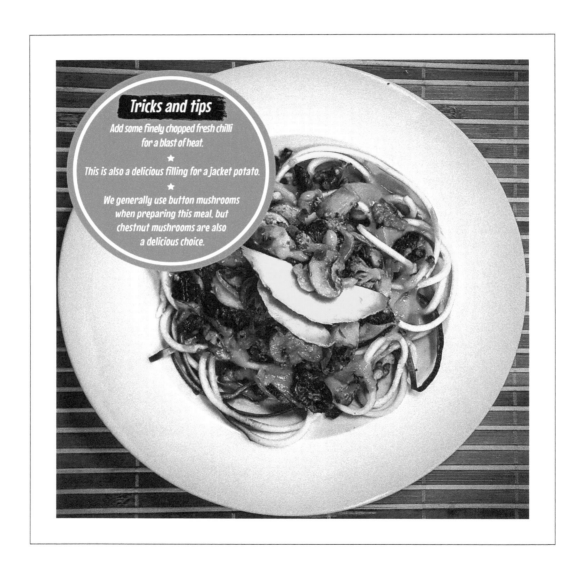

Tricks and tips

Add some finely chopped fresh chilli for a blast of heat.

★

This is also a delicious filling for a jacket potato.

★

We generally use button mushrooms when preparing this meal, but chestnut mushrooms are also a delicious choice.

D-Toxd mushroom Alfredo

If you're craving a tasty, creamy 'pasta' dish, this is for you. It's a healthy take on a usually calorie-laden recipe. They key is to make sure your mushrooms are cooked to perfection (not soggy).

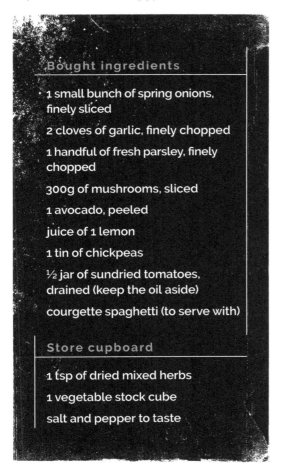

Bought ingredients

1 small bunch of spring onions, finely sliced

2 cloves of garlic, finely chopped

1 handful of fresh parsley, finely chopped

300g of mushrooms, sliced

1 avocado, peeled

juice of 1 lemon

1 tin of chickpeas

½ jar of sundried tomatoes, drained (keep the oil aside)

courgette spaghetti (to serve with)

Store cupboard

1 tsp of dried mixed herbs

1 vegetable stock cube

salt and pepper to taste

Putting it together

★ In a frying pan, lightly heat about 2 tbsp of the oil from the sundried tomatoes. Add the spring onions, garlic, parsley, mixed herbs, and vegetable stock cube and stir until the stock cube is dissolved and the spring onions are soft.

★ Add half the mushrooms and stir for two to three minutes (until they're well coated and slightly cooked — don't cook them too long or they'll go soggy).

★ Place the avocado, lemon juice, chickpeas (with the juice from the tin) and a few sundried tomatoes into a blender and blend until smooth — if the mixture is too thick, add a little water; it should have a creamy consistency.

★ Add to the mushroom mix and stir.

★ Chop up the remaining sundried tomatoes, add to the mixture with your remaining mushrooms, and cook for five minutes (until everything is nicely heated and well mixed). Season to taste and serve with courgette spaghetti.

D-Toxd chilli sin carne

Our take on this timeless classic is easy to prepare, warming, and totally delicious. Make it the day before you eat it and the flavours will be even better.

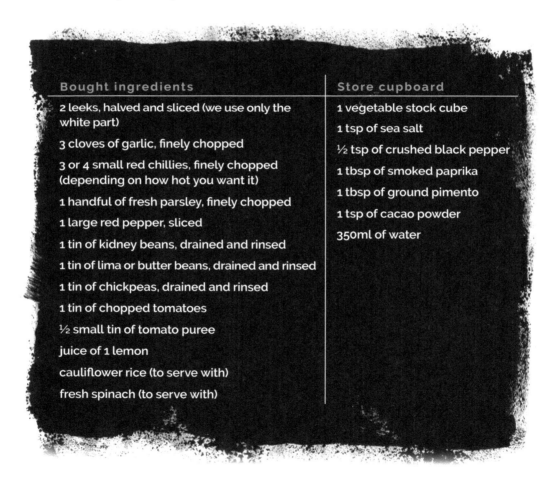

Bought ingredients

2 leeks, halved and sliced (we use only the white part)

3 cloves of garlic, finely chopped

3 or 4 small red chillies, finely chopped (depending on how hot you want it)

1 handful of fresh parsley, finely chopped

1 large red pepper, sliced

1 tin of kidney beans, drained and rinsed

1 tin of lima or butter beans, drained and rinsed

1 tin of chickpeas, drained and rinsed

1 tin of chopped tomatoes

½ small tin of tomato puree

juice of 1 lemon

cauliflower rice (to serve with)

fresh spinach (to serve with)

Store cupboard

1 vegetable stock cube

1 tsp of sea salt

½ tsp of crushed black pepper

1 tbsp of smoked paprika

1 tbsp of ground pimento

1 tsp of cacao powder

350ml of water

Putting it together

★ In a large saucepan, lightly steam-fry the leeks, garlic, chillies, parsley (keep some aside to garnish at the end), stock cube, salt, and pepper with a small amount of water (until the leeks are soft and the stock cube has dissolved).

★ Add the red pepper, paprika, and pimento and mix until well blended.

★ Add the beans and chickpeas. Stir until everything is coated with the leek and spice mixture.

★ Pour in tinned tomatoes and tomato puree and stir until well mixed.

★ Pour in water, stir, and let simmer for fifteen minutes. If it gets too thick, simply add more water.

★ Season to taste and mix through the lemon juice and cacao powder.

★ Serve with cauliflower rice (see Rocket FUEL) and fresh spinach and garnish with chopped parsley.

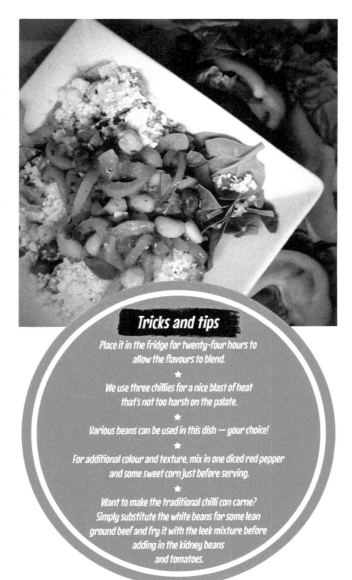

Tricks and tips

Place it in the fridge for twenty-four hours to allow the flavours to blend.

★

We use three chillies for a nice blast of heat that's not too harsh on the palate.

★

Various beans can be used in this dish — your choice!

★

For additional colour and texture, mix in one diced red pepper and some sweet corn just before serving.

★

Want to make the traditional chilli con carne? Simply substitute the white beans for some lean ground beef and fry it with the leek mixture before adding in the kidney beans and tomatoes.

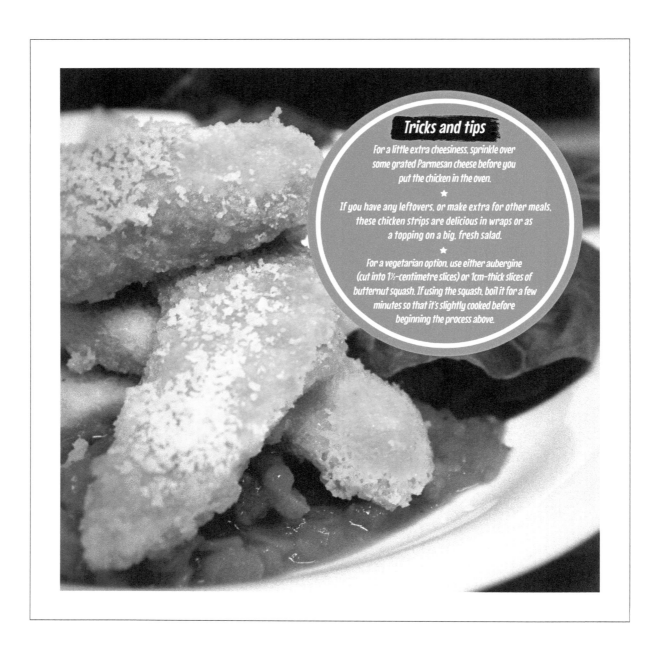

Tricks and tips

For a little extra cheesiness, sprinkle over some grated Parmesan cheese before you put the chicken in the oven.

★

If you have any leftovers, or make extra for other meals, these chicken strips are delicious in wraps or as a topping on a big, fresh salad.

★

For a vegetarian option, use either aubergine (cut into 1½-centimetre slices) or 1cm-thick slices of butternut squash. If using the squash, boil it for a few minutes so that it's slightly cooked before beginning the process above.

Grilled Parmesan chicken

Move over crumbed chicken because these chicken strips are tender, tasty, and packed full of protein. We serve this with steamed vegetables and the delicious smoked paprika and garlic tomato sauce.

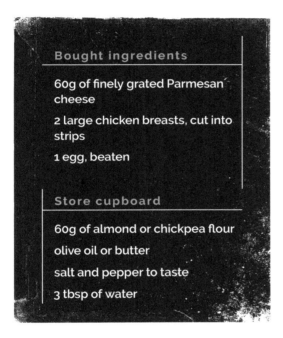

Bought ingredients

60g of finely grated Parmesan cheese

2 large chicken breasts, cut into strips

1 egg, beaten

Store cupboard

60g of almond or chickpea flour

olive oil or butter

salt and pepper to taste

3 tbsp of water

Putting it together

★ Preheat oven to 150 degrees Celsius.

★ Leaving aside two to three tbsp of flour, mix the cheese and flour until well blended.

★ Dust the chicken strips with the remaining flour until lightly coated.

★ Beat the egg and water together until well mixed.

★ Dip the chicken strips into the egg mixture and then into the cheese mixture, making sure the coating is even and thick.

★ In a frying pan, lightly heat the olive oil or butter and gently fry the chicken pieces so that they're nicely sealed. This will take only two to three minutes on each side (the aim is to seal them with a nice golden-brown colour and not to cook them through).

★ Place on a baking tray lined with greaseproof paper, cover with foil, and bake them slowly in the oven for fifteen to twenty minutes so that they remain nice and juicy.

★ Season to taste.

Smoked paprika and garlic tomato sauce

This smoky, tangy sauce is the ideal companion for the grilled Parmesan chicken but can also be used as a pasta sauce.

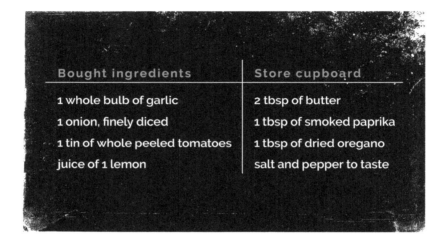

Bought ingredients	Store cupboard
1 whole bulb of garlic	2 tbsp of butter
1 onion, finely diced	1 tbsp of smoked paprika
1 tin of whole peeled tomatoes	1 tbsp of dried oregano
juice of 1 lemon	salt and pepper to taste

Putting it together

★ Preheat oven to 180 degrees Celsius.

★ Slice the top off the head of garlic and press half the butter into it. Wrap it in tinfoil so that it's a nicely sealed parcel and bake for about thirty minutes.

★ Using a medium-sized saucepan, fry the onion with the remaining butter (until it's soft and golden brown). Keep stirring it so that it doesn't catch.

* Add the tomatoes, smoked paprika, and oregano and cook on low heat for about ten minutes. If the mixture goes too dry, add a little water.

* Remove garlic from the oven and squeeze out the flesh straight into the sauce — when it's cooked, the garlic will have a creamy consistency and will come out easily when lightly squeezed.

* Mix and let simmer for five minutes on a low heat.

* Using a potato masher, mash the sauce until it's thick and chunky. Remember, if it's too thick, you can always add little water.

* Season with salt and pepper and stir in the lemon juice just before serving.

Tricks and tips

If you would rather use fresh tomatoes, place three or four large tomatoes into boiling water for about five minutes (doing so will make them easier to peel). Remove from the water and let cool, then peel and use as a substitute for the tinned tomatoes.

★

If using fresh tomatoes, you may need to add a tsp of brown sugar to the sauce to remove the slightly acidic taste fresh tomatoes can sometimes have once cooked.

★

For a bit of spice, add some freshly chopped chilli to your sauce during cooking.

Lemon, bacon, and cherry-tomato baked cod

There's nothing better than a piece of fresh fish — and making sure it's fresh is half the battle when creating a delicious, healthy meal. It's best not to serve too many strong flavours with fish, so finding tastes that complement it is important. Keep the flavours fresh and light and the fish will do the work for you.

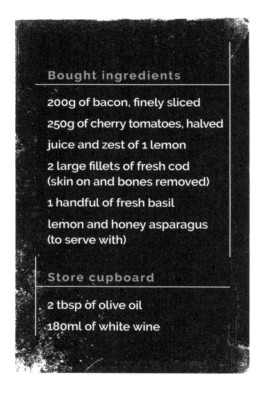

Bought ingredients

200g of bacon, finely sliced

250g of cherry tomatoes, halved

juice and zest of 1 lemon

2 large fillets of fresh cod
(skin on and bones removed)

1 handful of fresh basil

lemon and honey asparagus
(to serve with)

Store cupboard

2 tbsp of olive oil

180ml of white wine

Putting it together

★ Preheat oven to 160 degrees Celsius.

★ In a large pan, lightly heat the oil and fry the bacon until it begins to turn crispy and brown.

★ Throw in the cherry tomatoes and turn up the heat — you want them to reduce and get some colour, too.

★ Add the wine and lemon juice and zest, and continue cooking until the mixture has reduced by half.

★ Place the fish fillets in a well-greased oven dish and pour over the bacon and tomato mixture.

★ Cover with tinfoil and cook in the oven for about twenty minutes. You'll be able to tell if the fish is cooked by sticking a fork in the thickest part of the fillet — if cooked, the fish will still be moist and will flake easily.

★ Roughly tear up the fresh basil and sprinkle over the fish.

★ Serve with a side of lemon and honey asparagus (see Rocket FUEL).

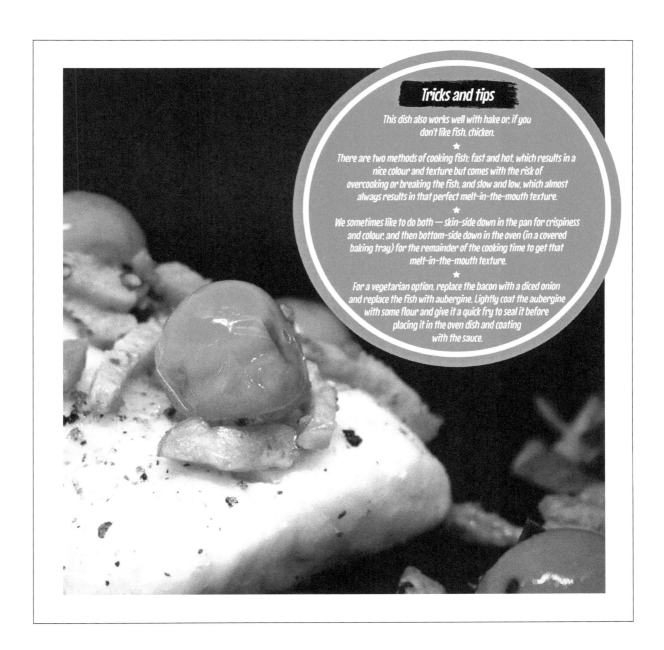

Tricks and tips

This dish also works well with hake or, if you don't like fish, chicken.

★

There are two methods of cooking fish: fast and hot, which results in a nice colour and texture but comes with the risk of overcooking or breaking the fish, and slow and low, which almost always results in that perfect melt-in-the-mouth texture.

★

We sometimes like to do both — skin-side down in the pan for crispiness and colour, and then bottom-side down in the oven (in a covered baking tray) for the remainder of the cooking time to get that melt-in-the-mouth texture.

★

For a vegetarian option, replace the bacon with a diced onion and replace the fish with aubergine. Lightly coat the aubergine with some flour and give it a quick fry to seal it before placing it in the oven dish and coating with the sauce.

Lentil cottage pie with mustard sweet potato mash

One of the most comforting meals in the book, this dish is best prepared in advance because when left to stand overnight, it takes on delicious earthy, smoky flavours. This does take a bit of advance planning, but it's ideal if you want leftovers for lunch or another dinner.

Bought ingredients	Store cupboard
1 onion, finely diced	25ml of olive oil
2 cloves of garlic, finely chopped	1 vegetable stock cube
1 handful of fresh parsley, finely chopped	1 tbsp of smoked paprika
3 large carrots, finely diced	1 tsp of ground pimento
1 red pepper, finely diced	1 tsp of curry powder
125g of dried red lentils	½ tsp of ground cumin
1 tin of chopped tomatoes	1 tbsp of wholegrain mustard
1 small tin of tomato puree	salt and pepper to taste
3 sweet potatoes, peeled, boiled, and mashed	50ml of water

Putting it together

★ On medium heat, lightly fry the onion, garlic, parsley, stock cube, and spices in the olive oil (until the onion is soft and everything is mixed together).

★ Add the carrots and stir for two to three minutes.

★ Add the red pepper and stir for two to three minutes.

★ Add the lentils and stir for about five minutes, until everything is coated. You can add a little water if the mixture is too dry.

- Mix in the tinned tomatoes and tomato puree and let simmer for a few minutes.

- Add water to just cover the mixture and bring to the boil while stirring.

- Turn the heat down and let simmer for ten to fifteen minutes, or until the lentils are almost cooked.

- Remove from heat, let cool, and place in the fridge overnight.

- The next day, heat on the stove for about twenty minutes (until lentils are nicely cooked). You may need to add a cup of water as the mixture can thicken during the night (this thickening and standing overnight is what brings out the smoky flavours).

- When heated through, place in baking tray and top with mashed sweet potato with the wholegrain mustard mixed through.

- Place under the grill for about fifteen minutes (until the top is golden brown and crispy).

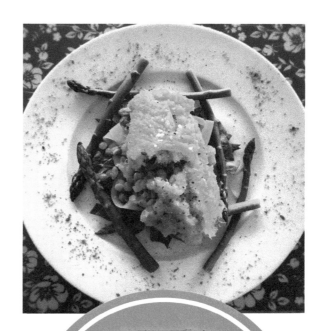

Tricks and tips

Depending on what lentils you use, the cooking time will vary. Check your mixture regularly as you don't want it to stick to the bottom of the pot.

★

Store any leftovers in containers and place in the freezer for use at a later date. This can stay in the freezer for up to a month, but we wouldn't keep it for longer than that.

Miripiri's beef stroganoff with a D-Toxd twist

We all love a homely, comforting stew, and this classic is just as delicious without the dairy. The blended chickpeas give it a rich, smooth taste. This recipe was kindly contributed by a close friend of D-Toxd.

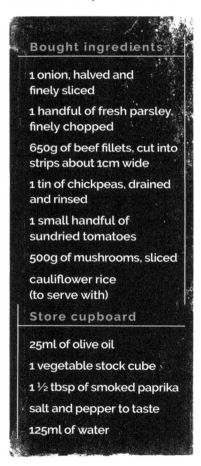

Bought ingredients

1 onion, halved and finely sliced

1 handful of fresh parsley, finely chopped

650g of beef fillets, cut into strips about 1cm wide

1 tin of chickpeas, drained and rinsed

1 small handful of sundried tomatoes

500g of mushrooms, sliced

cauliflower rice (to serve with)

Store cupboard

25ml of olive oil

1 vegetable stock cube

1 ½ tbsp of smoked paprika

salt and pepper to taste

125ml of water

Putting it together

★ Lightly heat the olive oil in a large saucepan and gently fry the stock cube, onion, and half the parsley (until the stock cube is dissolved and the onion is golden brown but not browned).

★ Add the smoked paprika and mix for about one minute (until well combined).

★ Toss in the fillets and cook until brown, adding a small amount of water if the mixture gets too dry and starts sticking. This will probably take about five minutes.

★ In a blender, blend the chickpeas and sundried tomatoes with the water until very smooth (about two to three minutes).

★ Pour the mixture into the saucepan and stir well, bringing it to the boil. If it's a little thick, add a splash more water.

★ Reduce the heat and let simmer for ten to fifteen minutes, stirring regularly.

★ Add the mushrooms and mix them through, cover, and let simmer for another five minutes.

★ Season to taste, serve with cauliflower rice (see Rocket FUEL), and garnish with the remaining parsley.

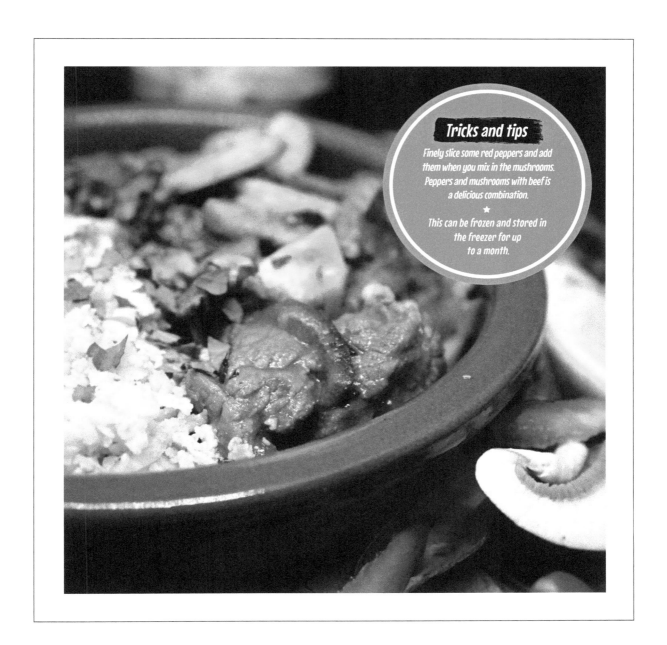

Tricks and tips

Finely slice some red peppers and add them when you mix in the mushrooms. Peppers and mushrooms with beef is a delicious combination.

★

This can be frozen and stored in the freezer for up to a month.

Oven-baked sea bass with sweet potato chilli mash

There's nothing better than an easy-to-prepare dish full of flavour and goodness. This is one of those dishes. Simply sit back, relax, and wait for it to be ready.

Bought ingredients	Store cupboard
2 sea bass fillets (skin on and bones removed)	2 tbsp of solid coconut oil
1 red onion, halved and finely sliced	1 tbsp of butter
2 cloves of garlic, finely sliced	¼ tsp of ground cinnamon
1 handful of fresh parsley, finely chopped	salt and pepper to taste
1 or 2 red chillies, finely sliced	
2 or 3 sweet potatoes, peeled and cubed	
2 handfuls of fresh spinach, finely chopped	

Putting it together

★ Preheat oven to 220 degrees Celsius and line a baking tray with greaseproof paper.

★ Place the fish on the baking tray and coat with the coconut oil.

★ Sprinkle over the onion, garlic, parsley, and half the chillies, season lightly, and place in the oven for twenty minutes, or until the fish is cooked. You'll be able to tell if it's cooked by sticking a fork in the thickest part of the fillet — if it's cooked, the fish will still be moist and will flake easily.

★ While the fish is baking, boil the sweet potatoes in slightly salted water (until they're tender and cooked through).

★ Drain and return to the saucepan, add the butter, and mash until smooth. Stir through the remaining chilli and cinnamon until well mixed.

★ Serve the mashed sweet potato on the spinach and top with the baked fish.

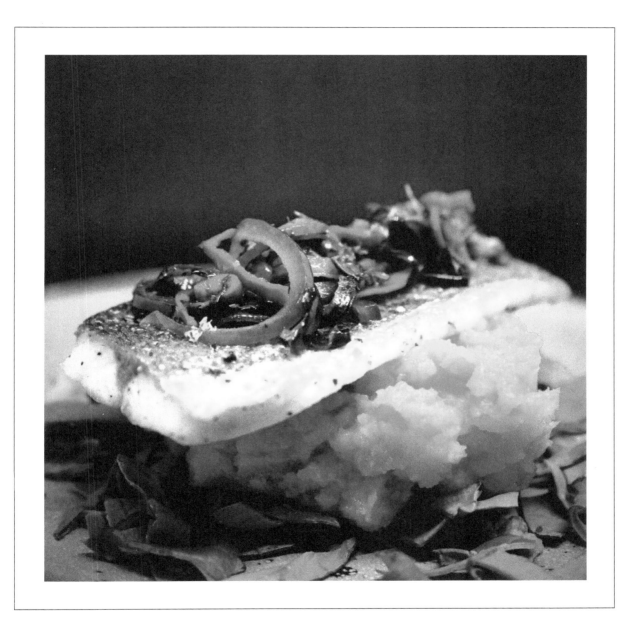

Pumpkin and pea risotto

Delicious comfort food, ideal for a chilly evening. The trick to a nice, creamy risotto is to keep stirring, to make sure the rice soaks up all the juices.

Bought ingredients	Store cupboard
1 onion, finely diced	1 tbsp of butter
2 cloves of garlic, finely chopped	1 tbsp of olive oil
1 handful of fresh parsley, finely chopped	125ml of white wine
250g of mixed wild rice	375ml of vegetable stock
125g of butternut squash, diced	salt and pepper to taste
1 handful of mushrooms, chopped	
125g of fresh or frozen peas	
60g of Parmesan cheese	
fresh spinach, finely chopped	

Putting it together

★ Heat half the butter and all the olive oil in a pot and gently cook the onion, garlic, and three quarters of the parsley (until the onions are soft and golden).

★ Add the rice and stir well until nicely coated.

★ Add half the wine and stir well for about three or four minutes (so that the wine reduces and the rice soaks it up).

★ Add the remaining wine once the previous wine has reduced; repeat the stirring process.

★ Add the butternut squash and stir well until everything is nicely coated.

★ About half a cup at a time, add the vegetable stock and mix well. Stir often until all the mixture is absorbed — you don't want the liquid to be boiling but gently simmering.

★ With your last half-cup of vegetable stock, add the mushrooms and peas and mix well.

★ When the risotto is almost finished, add the cheese and the remaining parsley and butter. Mix well until nice and creamy. Serve with spinach on top.

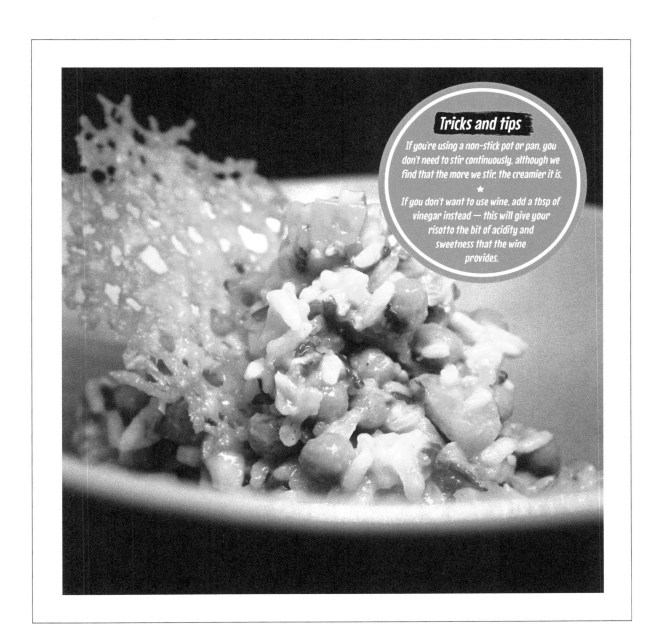

Tricks and tips

If you're using a non-stick pot or pan, you don't need to stir continuously, although we find that the more we stir, the creamier it is.

★

If you don't want to use wine, add a tbsp of vinegar instead — this will give your risotto the bit of acidity and sweetness that the wine provides.

Roast butternut squash and red pepper sauce

Butternut squash and red pepper are the perfect combination for a hearty, warming meal packed full of flavour and nutrients.

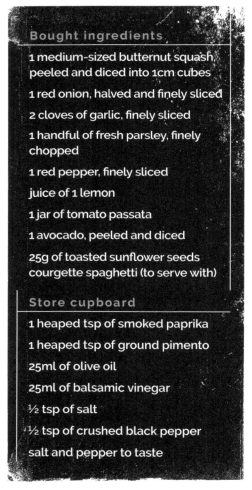

Bought ingredients

1 medium-sized butternut squash, peeled and diced into 1cm cubes

1 red onion, halved and finely sliced

2 cloves of garlic, finely sliced

1 handful of fresh parsley, finely chopped

1 red pepper, finely sliced

juice of 1 lemon

1 jar of tomato passata

1 avocado, peeled and diced

25g of toasted sunflower seeds
courgette spaghetti (to serve with)

Store cupboard

1 heaped tsp of smoked paprika

1 heaped tsp of ground pimento

25ml of olive oil

25ml of balsamic vinegar

½ tsp of salt

½ tsp of crushed black pepper

salt and pepper to taste

Putting it together

★ Preheat oven to 180 degrees Celsius.

★ Place squash, onion, garlic, parsley, and half the red pepper on a baking tray.

★ Cover with smoked paprika and ground pimento.

★ In a jug, mix the olive oil, balsamic vinegar, salt, pepper, lemon juice, and tomato passata and pour over vegetables.

★ Toss until everything is nicely coated and place on a lined baking tray.

★ Cover baking tray with tinfoil and bake for forty-five minutes to an hour.

★ Halfway though, remove baking tray and stir everything. If the mixture seems too dry, add a little water.

★ About ten minutes before serving, remove tray from oven and stir through remaining red pepper and the avocado, leaving about a quarter of the avocado aside.

★ Switch off oven and return tray for about ten minutes.

★ Serve with courgette spaghetti and sprinkle over remaining avocado and the sunflower seeds.

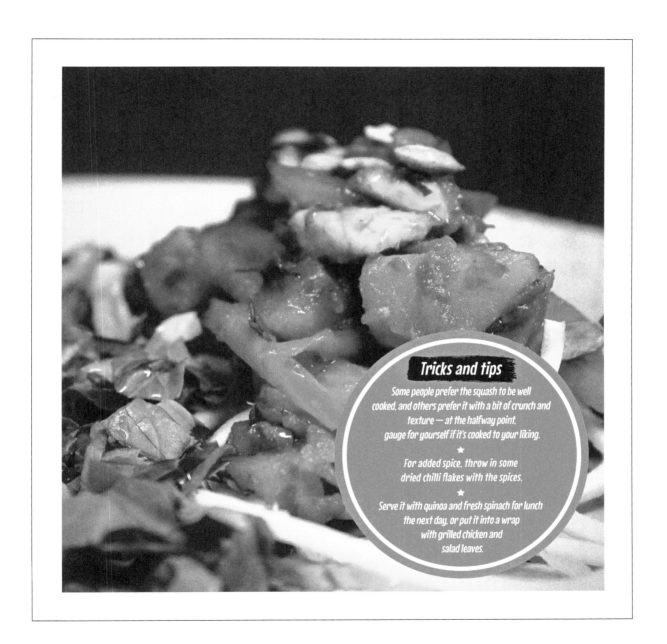

Tricks and tips

Some people prefer the squash to be well cooked, and others prefer it with a bit of crunch and texture — at the halfway point, gauge for yourself if it's cooked to your liking.

★

For added spice, throw in some dried chilli flakes with the spices.

★

Serve it with quinoa and fresh spinach for lunch the next day, or put it into a wrap with grilled chicken and salad leaves.

Roast fennel and onion with mushrooms, broccoli, and avocado cream

Many of the meals we prepare are the result of experiments that worked out well, including this one. We wanted something with a 'meaty' taste on a rainy day.

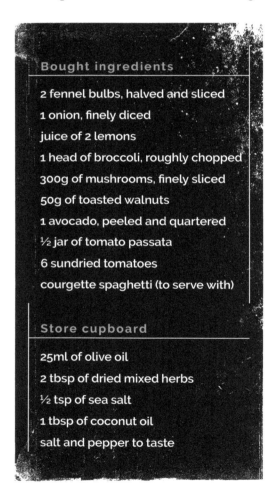

Bought ingredients

2 fennel bulbs, halved and sliced

1 onion, finely diced

juice of 2 lemons

1 head of broccoli, roughly chopped

300g of mushrooms, finely sliced

50g of toasted walnuts

1 avocado, peeled and quartered

½ jar of tomato passata

6 sundried tomatoes

courgette spaghetti (to serve with)

Store cupboard

25ml of olive oil

2 tbsp of dried mixed herbs

½ tsp of sea salt

1 tbsp of coconut oil

salt and pepper to taste

Putting it together

★ Preheat oven to 200 degrees Celsius and prepare a roasting tray by lining it with greaseproof paper.

★ In a large mixing bowl, combine the fennel and onion with the olive oil, juice of one lemon, and half the mixed herbs and toss until everything is nicely coated with the herbs.

★ Place in the roasting tray and bake for twenty-five to thirty minutes (until the fennel and onion are soft and tender but not too dry).

★ While the fennel and onion are roasting, lightly steam the broccoli (until it's tender but still has a bit of crunch to it).

★ In a large frying pan, lightly fry the sliced mushrooms, using a small amount of olive oil or water, and lightly season with sea salt and the remaining mixed herbs while frying. This shouldn't take more than three or four minutes, as you just want to lightly fry the mushrooms. Remove from the pan and set aside.

* Return the pan to the heat and add the coconut oil. Once the oil is heated, add the walnuts and sea salt and gently fry for three or four minutes (until the walnuts turn golden brown). Remove from pan and drain on paper towel to remove excess oil.

* When the fennel and onion are soft and tender, mix in the fried mushrooms and return to the oven for a further ten minutes, stirring once half way through.

* To make the avocado cream, add three quarters of the avocado to a blender with the juice of one lemon, the tomato passata, and the sundried tomatoes and blend until smooth and creamy. If the cream is too thick, add a splash of water.

* Serve with courgette spaghetti — place the fennel, onion, and mushroom mixture on top of the courgette, pour over a serving of the avocado cream, and sprinkle over the toasted walnuts and the remaining avocado.

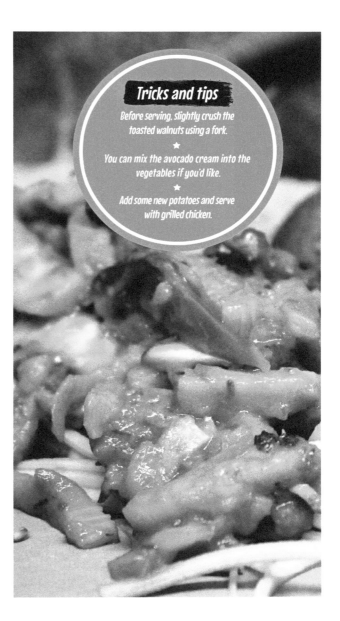

Tricks and tips

Before serving, slightly crush the toasted walnuts using a fork.

★

You can mix the avocado cream into the vegetables if you'd like.

★

Add some new potatoes and serve with grilled chicken.

Slow-baked butternut squash with courgette spaghetti

There are so many ways to cook butternut squash, and it's so good for you (and really tasty). The best thing about it? It's easy to cook and doesn't require much attention.

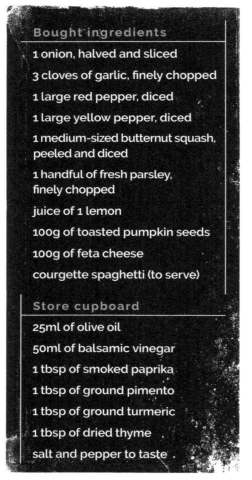

Bought ingredients

1 onion, halved and sliced

3 cloves of garlic, finely chopped

1 large red pepper, diced

1 large yellow pepper, diced

1 medium-sized butternut squash, peeled and diced

1 handful of fresh parsley, finely chopped

juice of 1 lemon

100g of toasted pumpkin seeds

100g of feta cheese

courgette spaghetti (to serve)

Store cupboard

25ml of olive oil

50ml of balsamic vinegar

1 tbsp of smoked paprika

1 tbsp of ground pimento

1 tbsp of ground turmeric

1 tbsp of dried thyme

salt and pepper to taste

Putting it together

★ Preheat oven to 180 degrees Celsius and line a baking tray with greaseproof paper.

★ In a large mixing bowl, combine all the ingredients except the pumpkin seeds and feta cheese and mix until everything is nicely coated. If you feel that you need more liquid, add a bit more lemon juice and balsamic vinegar (but remember that during the cooking, the pepper and onion will release some of their juices).

★ Bake for thirty to forty-five minutes. Check it every fifteen minutes or so to make sure that nothing is sticking. The trick with this recipe is to cook it slowly so that all the ingredients blend together.

★ Your squash should still be slightly firm at this point. Mix in the pumpkin seeds and return to the oven for another twenty minutes.

★ Once the squash is ready (it will be tender and the peppers will be soft), stir through the feta cheese and serve with courgette spaghetti. Don't mix it too much as the feta can break apart quite easily, and it's nice to have the chunks of cheesy texture with the dish.

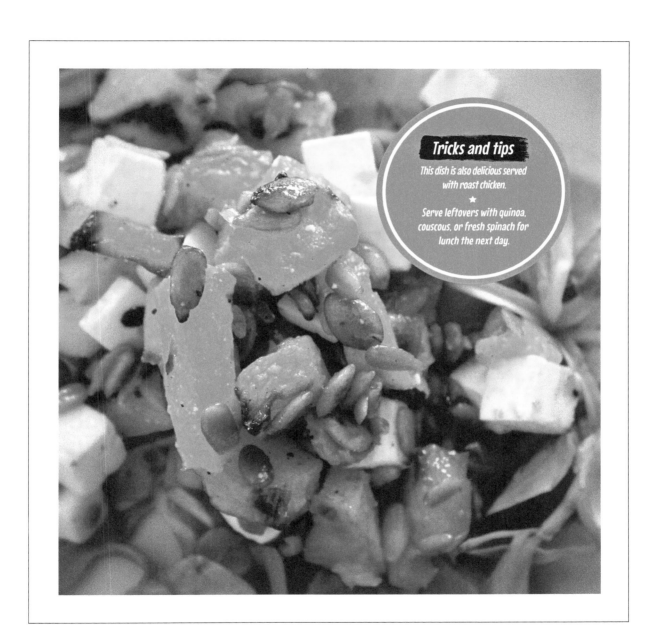

Tricks and tips

This dish is also delicious served with roast chicken.

★

Serve leftovers with quinoa, couscous, or fresh spinach for lunch the next day.

Stuffed red peppers

Red peppers are so tasty when slowly roasted, and when you combine them with more delicious vegetables, you don't need anything else to go with them.

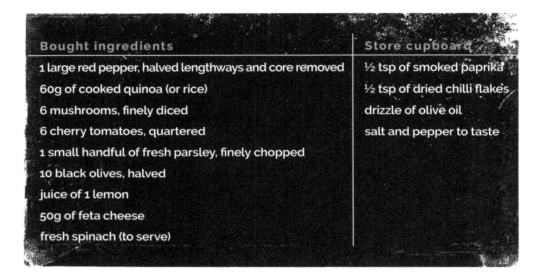

Bought ingredients	Store cupboard
1 large red pepper, halved lengthways and core removed	½ tsp of smoked paprika
60g of cooked quinoa (or rice)	½ tsp of dried chilli flakes
6 mushrooms, finely diced	drizzle of olive oil
6 cherry tomatoes, quartered	salt and pepper to taste
1 small handful of fresh parsley, finely chopped	
10 black olives, halved	
juice of 1 lemon	
50g of feta cheese	
fresh spinach (to serve)	

Putting it together

★ Preheat oven to 220 degrees Celsius and line a baking tray with greaseproof paper.

★ Place all the ingredients except for the red pepper halves in a mixing bowl and stir until everything is nicely mixed. Season to taste.

★ Spoon the filling into the peppers and pack down slightly.

★ Bake for about twenty to thirty minutes, or until the peppers are done. When it's ready, it will be soft and tender and the topping will have started to crisp and dry slightly.

★ Serve on a bed of fresh spinach with some of the Basic onion and tomato sauce (see Rocket FUEL.)

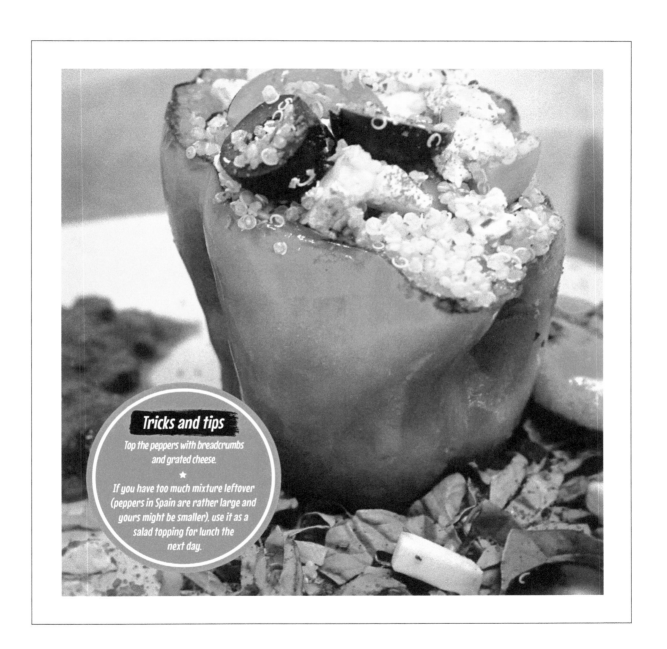

Tricks and tips

Top the peppers with breadcrumbs and grated cheese.

★

If you have too much mixture leftover (peppers in Spain are rather large and yours might be smaller), use it as a salad topping for lunch the next day.

Sweet potato and chickpea curry with fresh spinach

Sweet potatoes are packed with of goodness, and when you combine them with chickpeas and spinach, the result is a dish full of protein and flavour.

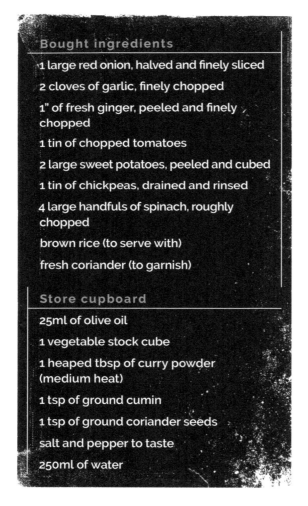

Bought ingredients

1 large red onion, halved and finely sliced

2 cloves of garlic, finely chopped

1" of fresh ginger, peeled and finely chopped

1 tin of chopped tomatoes

2 large sweet potatoes, peeled and cubed

1 tin of chickpeas, drained and rinsed

4 large handfuls of spinach, roughly chopped

brown rice (to serve with)

fresh coriander (to garnish)

Store cupboard

25ml of olive oil

1 vegetable stock cube

1 heaped tbsp of curry powder (medium heat)

1 tsp of ground cumin

1 tsp of ground coriander seeds

salt and pepper to taste

250ml of water

Putting it together

★ In a large saucepan, place the onion, garlic, ginger, oil, stock cube, and spices on medium heat. Stir until the onions are soft and golden brown and everything is nicely coated and mixed.

★ Add the tinned tomatoes and mix for two to three minutes, then add the sweet potatoes and mix well.

★ Pour in the water and bring to the boil, stirring so that it doesn't catch or stick to the bottom of the pot.

★ Reduce heat, cover, and simmer for ten to fifteen minutes (or until the sweet potato is cooked).

★ Pour in the chickpeas and stir to coat, then let simmer for another three to five minutes.

★ Remove the pot from the heat and mix through the spinach, allowing the residual heat to wilt the spinach.

★ Serve over a bed of brown rice and garnish with chopped coriander.

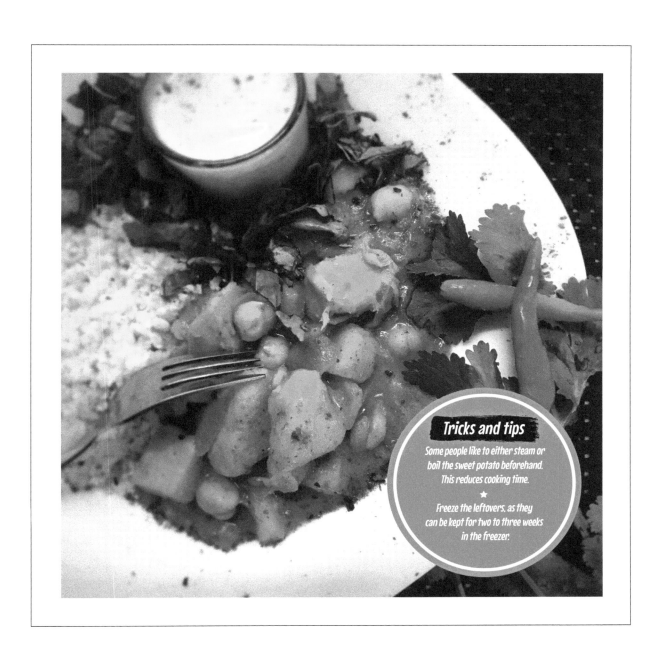

Tricks and tips

Some people like to either steam or boil the sweet potato beforehand. This reduces cooking time.

★

Freeze the leftovers, as they can be kept for two to three weeks in the freezer.

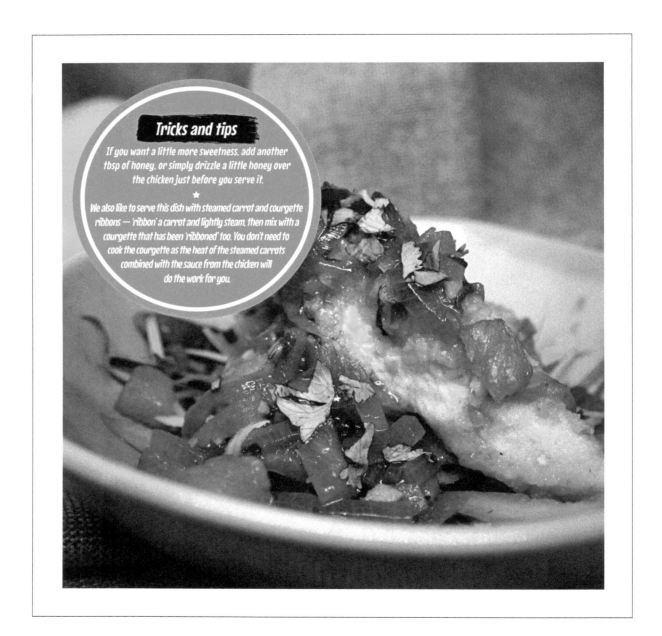

Tricks and tips

If you want a little more sweetness, add another tbsp of honey, or simply drizzle a little honey over the chicken just before you serve it.

★

We also like to serve this dish with steamed carrot and courgette ribbons — 'ribbon' a carrot and lightly steam, then mix with a courgette that has been 'ribboned' too. You don't need to cook the courgette as the heat of the steamed carrots combined with the sauce from the chicken will do the work for you.

Tangy sweet and spicy chicken

We love sweet and sour sauce, but we love a bit of spiciness even more. So we combined the three flavours! The combination of chilli and ginger is delicious.

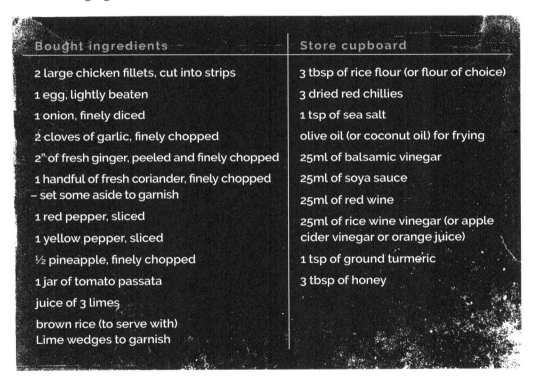

Bought ingredients	Store cupboard
2 large chicken fillets, cut into strips	3 tbsp of rice flour (or flour of choice)
1 egg, lightly beaten	3 dried red chillies
1 onion, finely diced	1 tsp of sea salt
2 cloves of garlic, finely chopped	olive oil (or coconut oil) for frying
2" of fresh ginger, peeled and finely chopped	25ml of balsamic vinegar
1 handful of fresh coriander, finely chopped – set some aside to garnish	25ml of soya sauce
1 red pepper, sliced	25ml of red wine
1 yellow pepper, sliced	25ml of rice wine vinegar (or apple cider vinegar or orange juice)
½ pineapple, finely chopped	1 tsp of ground turmeric
1 jar of tomato passata	3 tbsp of honey
juice of 3 limes	
brown rice (to serve with) Lime wedges to garnish	

Putting it together

★ Preheat oven to 180 degrees Celsius.

★ Place 2 tbsp of flour in a blender with the dried chillies and sea salt and blend well.

- ★ Lightly dust the chicken strips with the remaining flour, dip them in the egg, and then dip them in the seasoned flour, making sure they're lightly and evenly coated.

- ★ Heat olive oil in a frying pan and fry the strips for a few minutes on each side, until slightly golden. You don't want to fry the strips completely, just seal them. Once they're done, place in an ovenproof dish.

- ★ To prepare the sauce, fry the onion, garlic, ginger, turmeric and coriander in a small amount of oil until the onion and garlic are soft.

- ★ Add the peppers and pineapple and cook for five more minutes, stirring well so that the pineapple begins to reduce.

- ★ Add the tomato passata and let simmer for another five minutes before adding the lime juice, balsamic vinegar, soya sauce, red wine, rice vinegar, and honey.

- ★ Bring to the boil, reduce heat, and let simmer for ten minutes (until all the ingredients are soft and well cooked).

- ★ Spoon the cooked sauce over the top of the chicken, so that it's nicely covered (2 large serving spoons should do the trick.)

- ★ Cover the ovenproof dish with tinfoil and place in the oven for about twenty minutes, or until the chicken is cooked through, tender and juicy.

- ★ Remove from heat and serve with rice and more of the sauce poured over the top.

- ★ Garnish with fresh coriander and a lime wedge for added flavour.

Thai red curry paste

The health benefits of fresh, spicy food are endless, and Thai meals offer such a mixture of flavours. It's quick and easy to make your own curry paste.

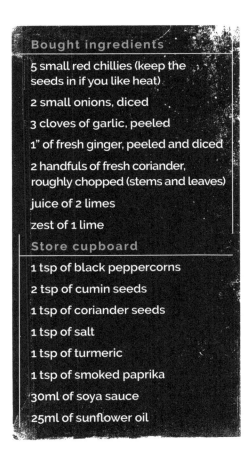

Bought ingredients

5 small red chillies (keep the seeds in if you like heat)

2 small onions, diced

3 cloves of garlic, peeled

1" of fresh ginger, peeled and diced

2 handfuls of fresh coriander, roughly chopped (stems and leaves)

juice of 2 limes

zest of 1 lime

Store cupboard

1 tsp of black peppercorns

2 tsp of cumin seeds

1 tsp of coriander seeds

1 tsp of salt

1 tsp of turmeric

1 tsp of smoked paprika

30ml of soya sauce

25ml of sunflower oil

Putting it together

★ Using a pestle and mortar, grind the peppercorns, cumin, and coriander seeds until fine.

★ Add all the ingredients to a blender and blend until it forms a thick paste. If it's too thick, add little bit of water or more oil.

★ Use with any of the delicious Thai dishes in the book. This paste will stay fresh in the fridge for a few weeks (as long as you keep it in an airtight container), and it can also be frozen.

Tricks and tips

You can use dried chillies instead of fresh ones — simply soak them for about ten minutes in hot water to let them soften.

★

If you want your paste to have more colour, soak a bit of saffron in a small amount of water for a few minutes and then add to the blend. Or simply add more paprika — for this recipe, we use sweet paprika rather than smoked.

★

You can use this paste with many different ingredients — vegetables, fish, chicken. Use your imagination and be creative.

Thai baked fish parcels

Baking food in parcels is similar to poaching or steaming, and allows all the flavours to combine during cooking.

Bought ingredients	Store cupboard
1 tsp of Thai red curry paste	1 tsp of corn flour
1 tin of coconut milk	25ml of soya sauce
1 tin of coconut cream	25ml of honey
juice of 2 limes	salt and pepper to taste
3 spring onions, finely sliced	
2 red chillies, finely sliced	
3 cloves of garlic, finely chopped	
1 handful of fresh coriander, roughly chopped	
2 large handfuls of baby spinach	
2 x 200g of white fish (we like to use cod or hake for this meal)	
steamed rice (to serve with)	
chopped coriander (to garnish)	
a few fine slices of chilli (to garnish)	

Putting it together

★ Preheat oven to 200 degrees Celsius.

★ Mix the flour with a little bit of coconut milk so that it forms a smooth mixture.

★ In a bowl, mix the curry paste, flour mixture, coconut milk, coconut cream, lime juice, onions, chillies, garlic, coriander, soya sauce, and honey until well blended.

- ★ Lay out two large pieces of tinfoil and then place two sheets of grease-proof paper on top of them — we like to lay them on large soup bowl as it gives us a shape to work with when creating the parcels.

- ★ Place a large handful of spinach in the middle of each parcel and press it down lightly — it might look like a lot of spinach, but it will wilt as it cooks.

- ★ Place a fish fillet on top of the spinach and turn up the sides of the foil parcel to form a bowl shape.

- ★ Pour half the sauce into each parcel and then scrunch the sides together so that the parcel is tightly sealed with all the deliciousness on the inside.

- ★ Bake for about fifteen to twenty minutes. You'll be able to tell if the fish is cooked by sticking a fork in the thickest part of the fillet — if cooked, the fish will still be moist and will flake easily.

- ★ To serve, open up the parcels and plate the fish on top of steamed rice. Pour over the remaining sauce and spinach from the parcel.

- ★ To garnish, sprinkle with coriander and chilli.

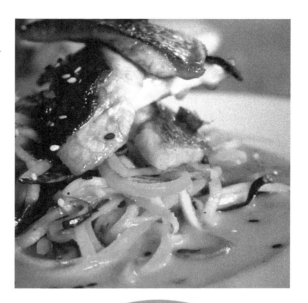

Tricks and tips

You can prepare this dish using prawns, chicken, or, for a vegetarian alternative, aubergine.

★

Clean prawns can be placed straight in, just like the fish.

★

When using chicken, we like to lightly seal it first, using a griddle pan on a high temperature — this gives it a slightly nicer texture and also a bit of colour.

★

When using aubergine, before baking, top and tail the vegetable then cut into quarters. Sprinkle with table salt and let stand for about thirty minutes — this brings out the moisture that can give aubergine a bitter taste. Pat it dry with paper towel and then, using a nice hot griddle pan, lightly fry it on all sides to give it some colour and texture.

Thai green vegetable curry

The flavours of Thai food work well with a wide variety of vegetables to give you dishes that are hard to resist. Even better? They're rather easy to make.

Green curry paste

Bought ingredients

1 tin of coconut milk

2 large handfuls of fresh coriander, leaves and stems

2 spring onions, roughly chopped

2 cloves of garlic, peeled

2 to 3 small green chillies (depending on how hot you want it)

1" of fresh ginger, peeled and roughly chopped

juice and zest of 1 lime

Store cupboard

salt and pepper to taste

½ cup of water

Curry

Bought ingredients

1 onion, finely diced

1" of fresh ginger, peeled and finely diced

1 red pepper, sliced

100g of baby corn, halved lengthways

100g of green beans or mangetout

1 cauliflower, roughly chopped
(use half for the curry and the other half to prepare cauliflower rice)

150g of mushrooms, finely sliced

1 portion of curry paste (as above)

1 courgette, halved and finely sliced

1 large carrot, finely sliced or taped
(use a potato peeler to get long ribbons)

1 large handful of broccoli florets

juice of 2 limes

cauliflower rice (to serve)

Store cupboard

25ml of coconut oil

3 tbsp of honey

25ml of soya sauce

salt and pepper to taste

Putting it together

★ To make the green curry paste, simply put all the ingredients into a blender and blend until smooth and creamy.

★ Lightly heat the oil and gently fry the onion and ginger until the onions are soft and tender.

★ Add the red pepper and baby corn and gently mix for two to three minutes (until everything is nicely coated).

★ Add the beans, cauliflower, half the mushrooms and three quarters of the curry paste and stir until everything is coated. Bring to the boil and let simmer for five minutes — the beans and cauliflower are slightly harder vegetables so need a bit of cooking time. If the mixture is too thick, add some water.

★ After five minutes, add the courgette, remaining mushrooms, carrot slices, and broccoli and let simmer for a further three or four minutes.

★ While the curry is simmering, mix together the remaining curry paste, lime juice, honey, and soya sauce then pour into the pot and mix everything.

★ Let simmer for a further five minutes.

★ Remove from heat and mix in the carrot ribbons — they'll give your curry a nice crunch. Cover and let stand for five minutes so that the curry's residual heat cooks the carrots.

★ Season to taste and serve with cauliflower rice (see Rocket FUEL).

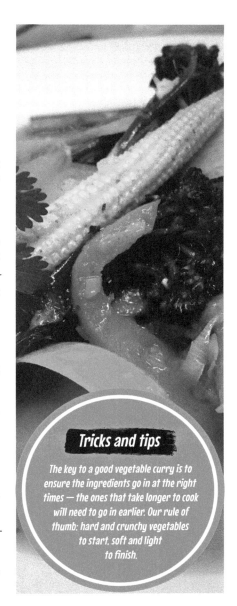

Tricks and tips

The key to a good vegetable curry is to ensure the ingredients go in at the right times — the ones that take longer to cook will need to go in earlier. Our rule of thumb: hard and crunchy vegetables to start, soft and light to finish.

Thai red vegetable curry

Bright. Bold. Quick. Easy.

Bought ingredients	Store cupboard
1 onion, finely diced	25ml of coconut oil
1 small red chilli, finely sliced	1 tsp of turmeric
2 cloves of garlic, finely chopped	25ml of soya sauce
1" of fresh ginger, peeled and finely chopped	3 tbsp of honey
1 handful of fresh coriander, finely chopped	salt and pepper to taste
½ butternut squash, peeled and diced	200ml of water
1 aubergine, diced	
2 tbsp of Thai red curry paste	
1 red pepper, sliced	
1 yellow pepper, sliced	
1 tin of coconut milk	
1 head of broccoli, roughly chopped	
juice of 1 lime	
3 large handfuls of fresh baby spinach	
cauliflower rice (to serve with)	
fresh coriander (to garnish)	
wedge of lime (to garnish)	

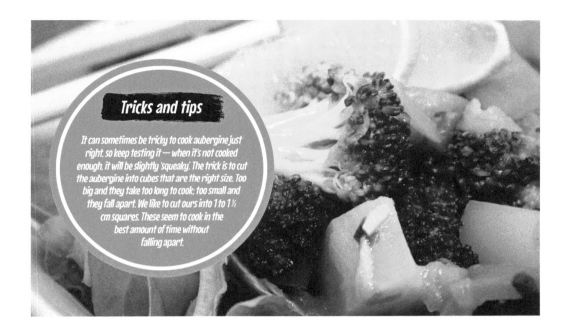

Tricks and tips

It can sometimes be tricky to cook aubergine just right, so keep testing it — when it's not cooked enough, it will be slightly 'squeaky'. The trick is to cut the aubergine into cubes that are the right size. Too big and they take too long to cook; too small and they fall apart. We like to cut ours into 1 to 1½ cm squares. These seem to cook in the best amount of time without falling apart.

Putting it together

★ In a large saucepan, lightly heat the coconut oil and gently fry the onion, chilli, garlic, ginger, turmeric, and half the coriander until the onions are soft and tender.

★ Add the squash, aubergine, and half the water, stir, and bring to the boil for two to three minutes, making sure the mixture isn't too dry.

★ Pour in the curry paste, red and yellow peppers, coconut milk, and soya sauce and mix well. Let simmer for five to ten minutes, stirring every three or four minutes.

★ Add the rest of the water and the honey and broccoli, then cover and simmer for another five minutes, or until the vegetables are cooked to your liking.

★ Remove from heat and stir through the lime juice and spinach. Cover and let stand for five minutes so that the residual heat of the curry cooks the spinach.

★ Season to taste and serve with rice noodles or cauliflower rice (see Rocket FUEL). Garnish with coriander and a wedge of lime.

Thai sweet potato curry

This version of sweet potato curry has an aromatic flavour with subtle hints of heat and sour.

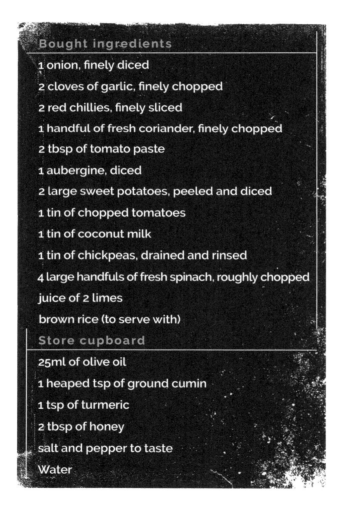

Bought ingredients

1 onion, finely diced

2 cloves of garlic, finely chopped

2 red chillies, finely sliced

1 handful of fresh coriander, finely chopped

2 tbsp of tomato paste

1 aubergine, diced

2 large sweet potatoes, peeled and diced

1 tin of chopped tomatoes

1 tin of coconut milk

1 tin of chickpeas, drained and rinsed

4 large handfuls of fresh spinach, roughly chopped

juice of 2 limes

brown rice (to serve with)

Store cupboard

25ml of olive oil

1 heaped tsp of ground cumin

1 tsp of turmeric

2 tbsp of honey

salt and pepper to taste

Water

Putting it together

★ In a large saucepan, lightly fry the olive oil, onion, garlic, chillies, half the coriander, and the spices until the onions are soft and golden brown.

★ Add the tomato paste and honey and mix well (no longer than a minute).

★ Add the aubergine and sweet potatoes and stir for two to three minutes.

★ Pour in the tomatoes, coconut milk and (using the tin from the coconut milk) one tin of water and bring to the boil, stirring regularly to ensure nothing sticks.

★ Once the curry is boiling, reduce heat and cover and cook for about thirty minutes, checking it regularly to make sure that nothing is catching.

* Add the chickpeas and half the spinach, mix well, and let simmer for another fifteen minutes. If the mixture is reducing too much, add more water. As the curry cooks, the sweet potatoes will break down and naturally thicken it; stirring it regularly will ensure it doesn't burn or catch.

* Check that the aubergine is cooked (it should be by this time) and remove from heat. Stir through the lime juice and remaining spinach and coriander and serve with brown rice.

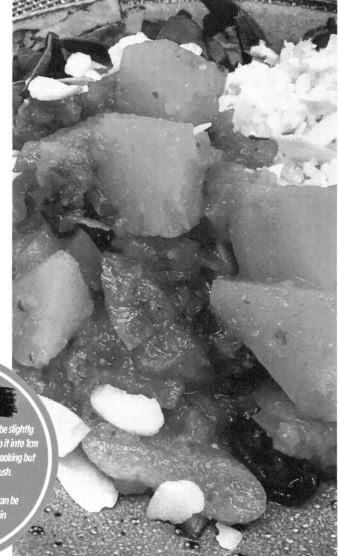

Tricks and tips

If aubergine doesn't cook properly, it will be slightly 'squeaky' when you eat it. The trick is to chop it into 1cm cubes: small enough to ensure thorough cooking but not so small that they'll turn to mush.

★

Leftovers can be frozen, or this dish can be prepared in advance and stored in airtight containers.

Tuna and apple wraps

A quick, easy, and refreshingly tasty meal packed full of nutrients.

Bought ingredients	Store cupboard
1 tin of tuna in brine, drained	1 tsp of wholegrain mustard
1 tbsp of Greek yogurt	1 tsp of honey
1 apple, diced	salt and pepper to taste
1 stick of celery, finely sliced	
juice of ½ lemon	
2 wholemeal wraps	
1 handful of baby spinach	
1 tomato, sliced	

Putting it together

★ In a bowl, mix the tuna, yogurt, apple, celery, lemon juice, mustard, and honey.

★ Place the wraps on a flat surface and divide the spinach leaves and tomato slices between the two wraps.

★ Spread half the mixture onto each wrap and season to taste.

★ Roll the wraps and enjoy.

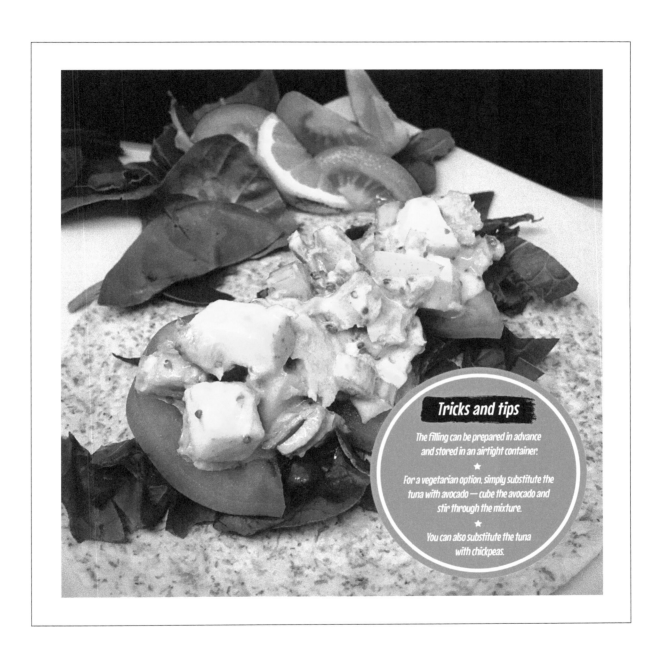

Tricks and tips

The filling can be prepared in advance
and stored in an airtight container.

★

For a vegetarian option, simply substitute the
tuna with avocado — cube the avocado and
stir through the mixture.

★

You can also substitute the tuna
with chickpeas.

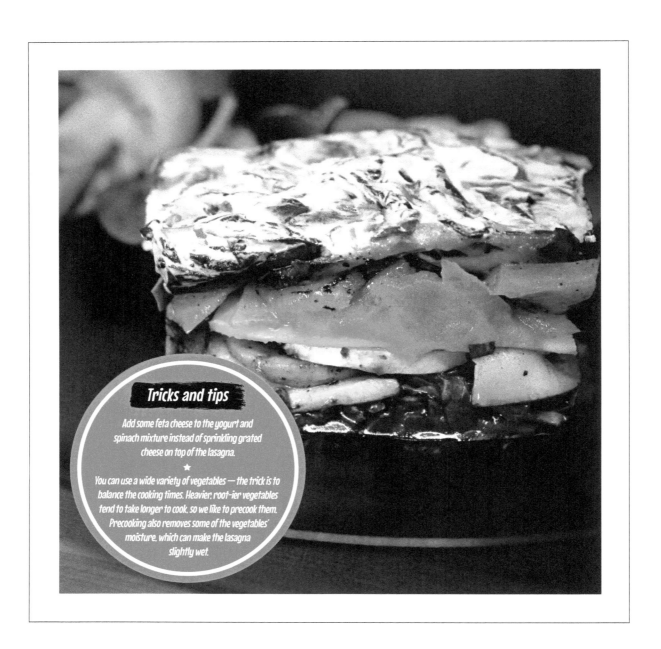

Tricks and tips

Add some feta cheese to the yogurt and spinach mixture instead of sprinkling grated cheese on top of the lasagna.

★

You can use a wide variety of vegetables — the trick is to balance the cooking times. Heavier, root-ier vegetables tend to take longer to cook, so we like to precook them. Precooking also removes some of the vegetables' moisture, which can make the lasagna slightly wet.

Vegetable lasagne

For this recipe, you can use vegetables of your choice and layer them as you wish. At D-Toxd, we use aubergine or courgette as our 'pasta'. Preparing the vegetables is time consuming, but the result is delicious, and this dish is great if you want leftovers. The quantities will vary, depending on the size of your baking dish.

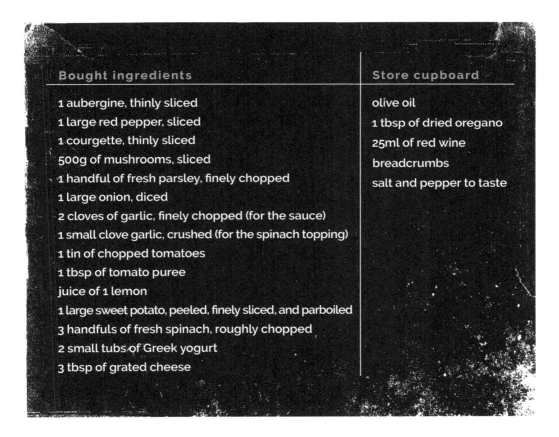

Bought ingredients	Store cupboard
1 aubergine, thinly sliced	olive oil
1 large red pepper, sliced	1 tbsp of dried oregano
1 courgette, thinly sliced	25ml of red wine
500g of mushrooms, sliced	breadcrumbs
1 handful of fresh parsley, finely chopped	salt and pepper to taste
1 large onion, diced	
2 cloves of garlic, finely chopped (for the sauce)	
1 small clove garlic, crushed (for the spinach topping)	
1 tin of chopped tomatoes	
1 tbsp of tomato puree	
juice of 1 lemon	
1 large sweet potato, peeled, finely sliced, and parboiled	
3 handfuls of fresh spinach, roughly chopped	
2 small tubs of Greek yogurt	
3 tbsp of grated cheese	

Putting it together

★ Preheat oven to 200 degrees Celsius.

★ Place aubergine, red pepper, and courgette on a baking tray and bake for ten to fifteen minutes (until vegetables are lightly grilled).

★ In a large saucepan, lightly fry the mushrooms with a small amount of parsley and a drop of olive oil until the mushrooms are slightly cooked and coated. Remove from pan and set aside.

★ Using the same pan, lightly steam-fry the onions, garlic, dried oregano, and parsley with some olive oil and stir until onions are golden brown. Pour in a splash of red wine and reduce while stirring.

★ Add the tinned tomatoes and bring to the boil. Reduce the heat and then simmer for four to five minutes, adding the tomato puree and lemon juice once this is done. Mix thoroughly.

★ Spoon some of the tomato mixture onto the base of an ovenproof dish and then layer the vegetables in the order of your choice. We generally layer as follows: tomato mixture, red pepper, aubergine, courgette, mushrooms, tomato mixture, sweet potato, aubergine, tomato, courgette, mushrooms (as you can see, there's no specific order).

★ Lightly fry the spinach with the crushed garlic (if you don't want to use oil, try a small amount of lemon juice; the spinach will wilt and release its own juices). Once the spinach has wilted, mix in a small tub of Greek yogurt and then layer on top.

★ Sprinkle some cheese and breadcrumbs on top and bake for about fifteen or twenty minutes (in preheated oven, same temperature as before), until the top is golden brown. Remember, most of the vegetables are already cooked, so just heat everything through and brown the top.

Basic onion and tomato sauce

This recipe makes about 700ml of sauce, which is enough for four meals.

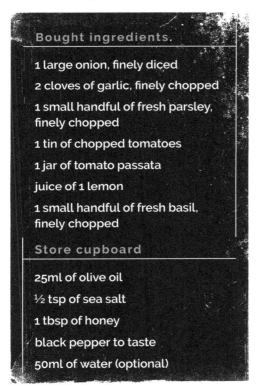

Bought ingredients.

1 large onion, finely diced

2 cloves of garlic, finely chopped

1 small handful of fresh parsley, finely chopped

1 tin of chopped tomatoes

1 jar of tomato passata

juice of 1 lemon

1 small handful of fresh basil, finely chopped

Store cupboard

25ml of olive oil

½ tsp of sea salt

1 tbsp of honey

black pepper to taste

50ml of water (optional)

Putting it together

★ In a saucepan, lightly heat the olive oil and gently fry the onion, garlic, parsley, and salt for about five minutes (until the onions are soft and tender).

★ Add the chopped tomatoes and honey and gently cook for another three or four minutes (until the tomatoes have reduced slightly).

★ Add the passata and lemon juice, bring to the boil, then reduce and simmer for about ten minutes, so that the mixture thickens. If you find your sauce is too thick, simply add a little water and reduce.

★ Mix through the fresh basil and season to taste.

★ If you like a smooth sauce, blend it once it's cooked and return to the stove and simmer for a few more minutes.

Cauliflower rice

This is a great substitute for rice, and is far healthier, too. It's simple to prepare and doesn't taste anything like cauliflower.

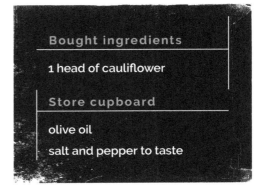

Bought ingredients

1 head of cauliflower

Store cupboard

olive oil

salt and pepper to taste

Putting it together

★ Roughly chop the cauliflower into chunks (excluding the centre stalk/thicker piece) and grate either by hand or using a food processor. If using a food processor, add a few chunks at a time and use the pulse button as you don't want it to break down too much and form a paste. It should have the consistency of large pieces of rice.

★ Heat a large frying pan and drizzle in a small amount of olive oil. Add 2 or 3 large handfuls of the grated cauliflower, season lightly, and gently mix with a wooden spoon. As the 'rice' fries, it will start to dry out and turn slightly golden; it will also become slightly fluffier.

★ Remove from the pan and continue in batches until all the cauliflower is fried (each batch will take about four or five minutes to cook).

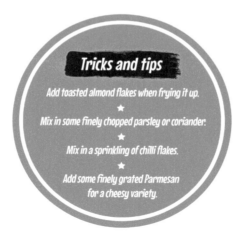

Tricks and tips

Add toasted almond flakes when frying it up.

★

Mix in some finely chopped parsley or coriander.

★

Mix in a sprinkling of chilli flakes.

★

Add some finely grated Parmesan for a cheesy variety.

D-Toxd green beans and spinach

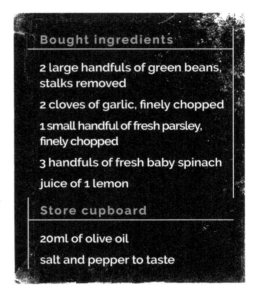

Bought ingredients

2 large handfuls of green beans, stalks removed

2 cloves of garlic, finely chopped

1 small handful of fresh parsley, finely chopped

3 handfuls of fresh baby spinach

juice of 1 lemon

Store cupboard

20ml of olive oil

salt and pepper to taste

Putting it together

★ Top and tail the green beans, slice them in half horizontally, then boil or steam until tender — you want them to be slightly crunchy.

★ Once the beans are done, heat the olive oil in a large pan, throw in the green beans, garlic, and parsley, and mix well, making sure the beans are well coated.

★ Add the spinach and lemon juice and toss until mixed.

★ Season to taste and serve.

Lemon and honey asparagus

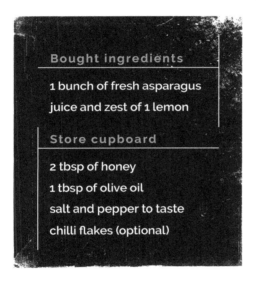

Bought ingredients

1 bunch of fresh asparagus

juice and zest of 1 lemon

Store cupboard

2 tbsp of honey

1 tbsp of olive oil

salt and pepper to taste

chilli flakes (optional)

Putting it together

★ Remove the bottoms of the asparagus and cut the stalks in half.

★ Lightly steam or boil the stalks but only for a few minutes — you want them to be a little firm.

★ In a small saucepan, mix the lemon juice and zest, honey, and olive oil and stir well until heated through to form a slightly thick sauce.

★ Remove from heat and throw in the cooked asparagus, stirring gently to coat.

★ Season to taste and serve.

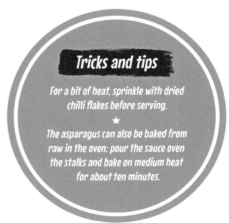

Tricks and tips

For a bit of heat, sprinkle with dried chilli flakes before serving.

★

The asparagus can also be baked from raw in the oven: pour the sauce oven the stalks and bake on medium heat for about ten minutes.

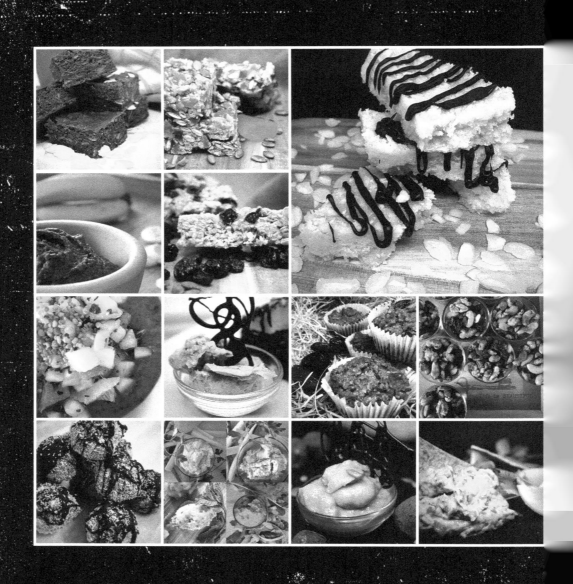

THE GUILT-FREE ZONE:
SNACKS, TREATS, AND DESSERTS
DONE THE FUEL WAY

We all deserve sweets and treats. Let's face it — at the end of the day, sometimes there's nothing better than sitting down with a nice cup of tea and a sweet treat. But that sweet treat doesn't have to be packed full of sugar and highly processed.

The Guilt-Free Zone is packed full of recipes to satisfy your sweet-tooth cravings and leave you feeling mischievous but totally (as the name says) guilt-free. Naughty doesn't come into it when you're living the FUEL way!

Then there are those times when you don't quite know what you want and aren't really hungry enough for a full meal. Having a few ideas for quick and easy snacks can mean the difference between reaching for a chocolate bar and reaching for something just as tasty but way better for you.

Recipes in this section

SNACKS, TREATS, AND DESSERTS

Apricot energy bar

Avocado and basil panna cotta

Avocado and pistachio ice cream

Banana ice cream

Birdseed bars

Caramel sauce

Chocolate fudge

Chocolate fudge cake

Chocolate hummus

Coconut delight

Courgette and almond brownies

Courgette and apple muffins

Cranberry granola bar

D-Toxd fruit salad and yogurt

D-Toxd hummus

D-Toxd mixed nuts and fruit

D-Toxd Peanut Butter bars

Energy balls

Quick and easy guacamole

Snacks, Treats, and Desserts

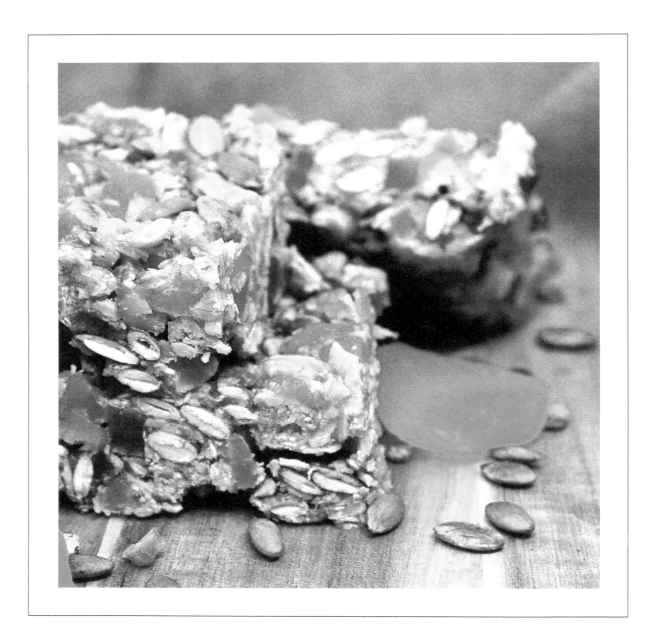

Apricot energy bar

Bought ingredients	Store cupboard
100g of dried apricots, roughly chopped	200ml of dissolved coconut oil
100g of flaked almonds	1 tbsp of ground ginger
100g of toasted pumpkin seeds	2 tbsp of honey
100g of dried oats	
100g of walnuts, roughly chopped	

Putting it together

★ In a large bowl, combine all ingredients and mix until everything is coated with the coconut oil.

★ Place on lined 20cm square baking tray and press down well.

★ Put in the fridge to set for two to three hours, then cut into squares and store in an airtight container.

Tricks and tips

The bars need to be stored in the fridge so that they remain firm. If you're taking them to work, wrap them in greaseproof paper and tinfoil so they keep well.

★

For added indulgence, sprinkle with cacao powder or drizzle with melted or grated dark chocolate before placing the mixture in the fridge to set.

★

You can add almost any dried fruit (eg. apple, ginger, kiwi fruit). The choice is up to you, but stick to unsweetened dried fruits that have not had highly processed sugars added to them — which are really not necessary, because when fruits are dried, their natural flavours are enhanced anyway.

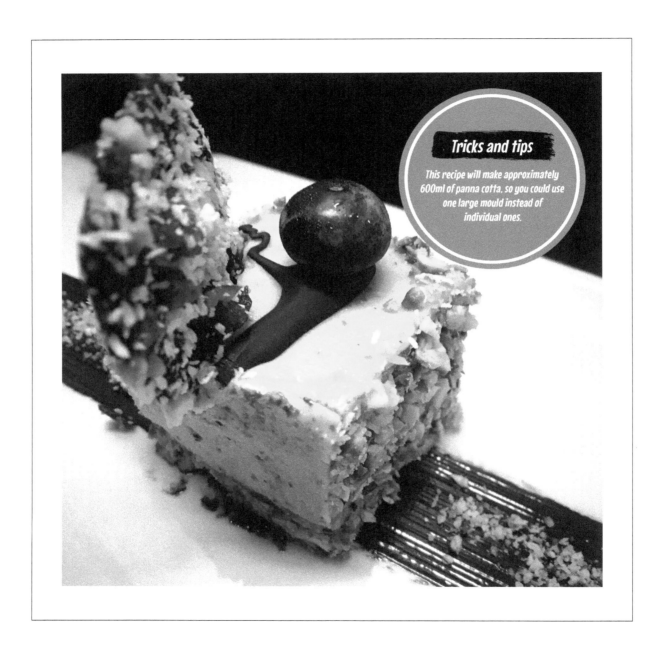

Tricks and tips

This recipe will make approximately 600ml of panna cotta, so you could use one large mould instead of individual ones.

Avocado and basil panna cotta

It might sound savoury, but this is definitely a refreshing, creamy sweet treat.

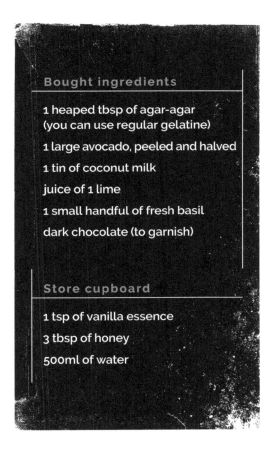

Bought ingredients

1 heaped tbsp of agar-agar
(you can use regular gelatine)

1 large avocado, peeled and halved

1 tin of coconut milk

juice of 1 lime

1 small handful of fresh basil

dark chocolate (to garnish)

Store cupboard

1 tsp of vanilla essence

3 tbsp of honey

500ml of water

★ In a small saucepan, prepare your agar-agar — we like to boil 500ml of water with 1 large tbsp. Boil for seven to eight minutes and then let cool. Make sure that all the agar-agar has dissolved; otherwise, you might end up with lumps (which aren't too nice).

★ Once the gelatine has cooled, place the avocado, coconut milk, lime juice, basil, vanilla, and honey into a food processor and blend for at least two minutes (until smooth and creamy).

★ Fill the coconut milk tin with the gelatine liquid and add to the coconut mixture while still blending. This will make it nice and fluffy and get rid of any lumps in the coconut milk or gelatine.

★ Place into moulds and store in the refrigerator for at least three or four hours (until set).

★ Unmould onto a plate and garnish with finely grated dark chocolate.

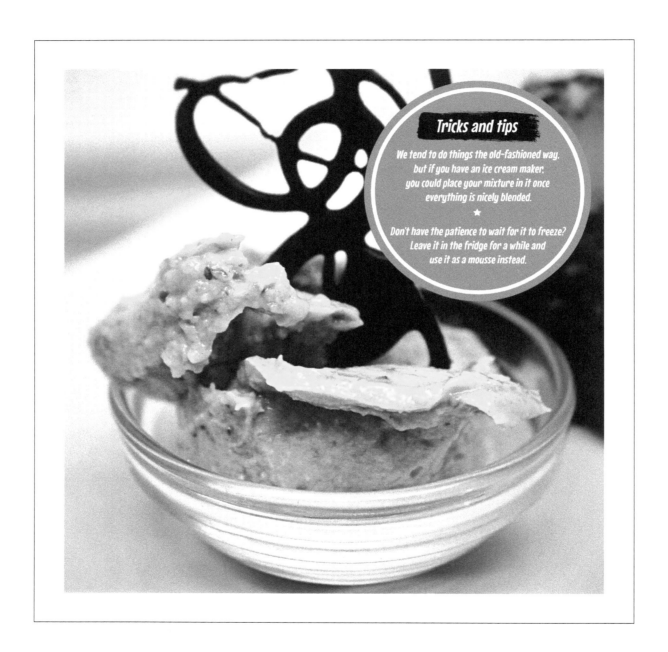

Tricks and tips

We tend to do things the old-fashioned way, but if you have an ice cream maker, you could place your mixture in it once everything is nicely blended.

★

Don't have the patience to wait for it to freeze? Leave it in the fridge for a while and use it as a mousse instead.

Avocado and pistachio ice cream

This dessert is simply delicious. There really are no other words for it. We wanted something that was full of goodness and health but still seemed slightly indulgent — this is what we came up with.

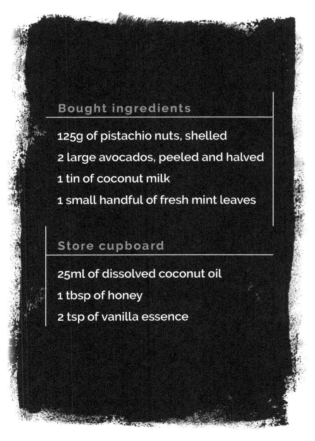

Bought ingredients

125g of pistachio nuts, shelled

2 large avocados, peeled and halved

1 tin of coconut milk

1 small handful of fresh mint leaves

Store cupboard

25ml of dissolved coconut oil

1 tbsp of honey

2 tsp of vanilla essence

Putting it together

★ Using a pestle and mortar, crush the pistachio nuts until they're roughly broken up (the size of breadcrumbs). Remove 1 large tbsp and set aside for use when serving.

★ Place all the ingredients into a food processor and blend until smooth and creamy. This will take at least four to five minutes.

★ Freeze in a large mixing bowl for at least four or five hours — every thirty to forty-five minutes, remove it from the freezer and mix it well.

★ When serving, garnish with the remaining pistachio nuts.

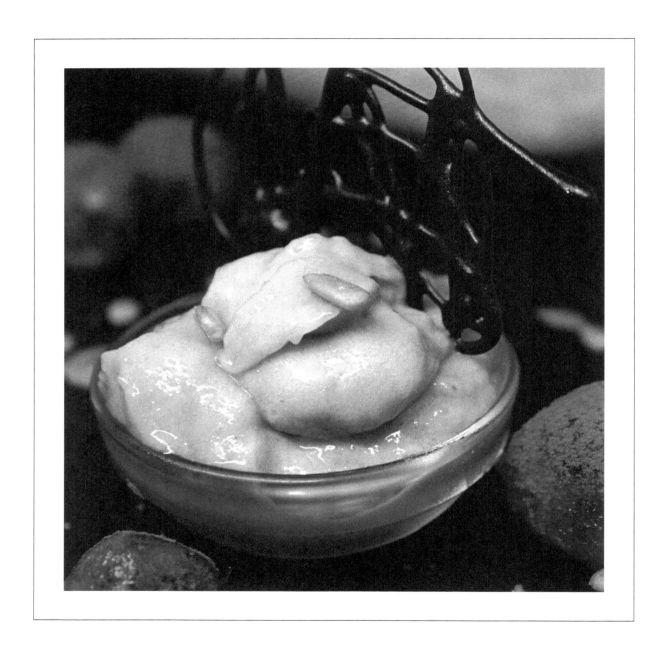

Banana ice cream

So quick and easy — the hardest part about this recipe is waiting for the bananas to freeze!

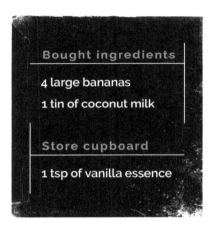

Bought ingredients

4 large bananas
1 tin of coconut milk

Store cupboard

1 tsp of vanilla essence

Putting it together

★ Peel and chop the bananas and freeze them in a plastic bag in the freezer (until frozen solid).

★ Place the tin of coconut milk in the freezer for about forty-five minutes (until it's well chilled and partially frozen).

★ Place all ingredients in the food processor and blend until smooth.

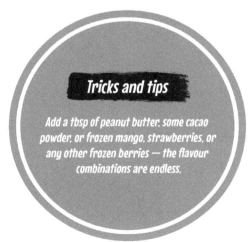

Tricks and tips

Add a tbsp of peanut butter, some cacao powder, or frozen mango, strawberries, or any other frozen berries — the flavour combinations are endless.

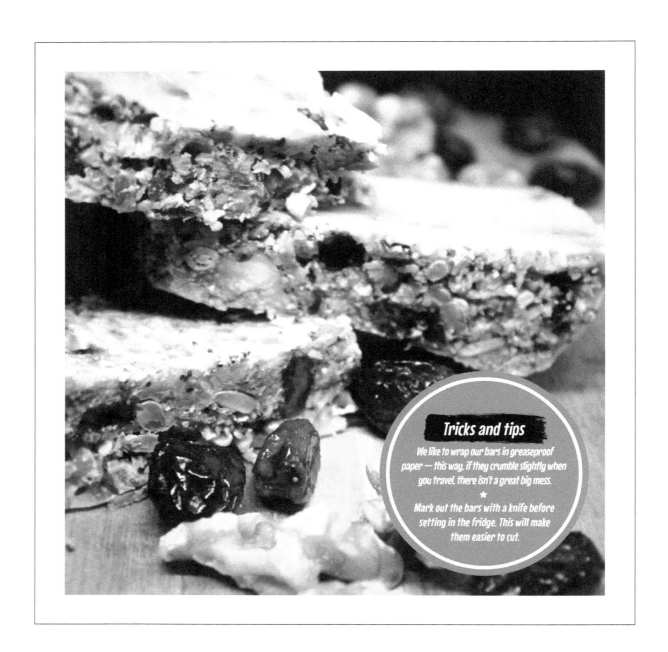

Tricks and tips

We like to wrap our bars in greaseproof paper — this way, if they crumble slightly when you travel, there isn't a great big mess.

★

Mark out the bars with a knife before setting in the fridge. This will make them easier to cut.

Birdseed bars

A tasty snack when you're feeling peckish. We get about sixteen bars from this recipe.

Bought ingredients	Store cupboard
125g of toasted sesame seeds	125ml of dissolved coconut oil
125g of toasted sunflower seeds	60ml of honey
125g of toasted walnuts, roughly chopped	1 tbsp of tahini
125g of desiccated coconut	1 tsp of vanilla essence
125g of cranberries	

Putting it together

★ Combine all the dry ingredients in a large mixing bowl and toss until well blended.

★ Melt together the coconut oil, honey, tahini, and vanilla essence, and then pour over the dried ingredients and mix well. Ensure everything is nicely coated with the oil and honey mixture.

★ Spread onto a flat baking tray (we use a 34cm x 20cm x 3cm tray) and let cool in the fridge for about an hour. The coconut oil will hold the bars together as it sets.

★ Cut into pieces and store in an airtight container in a cool, dark place.

Caramel sauce

Everyone loves caramel sauce, and coming up with a natural alternative that wasn't sky high in processed sugar was fun! This is, quite simply, the healthiest naughty treat ever.

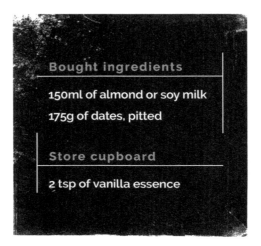

Bought ingredients

150ml of almond or soy milk

175g of dates, pitted

Store cupboard

2 tsp of vanilla essence

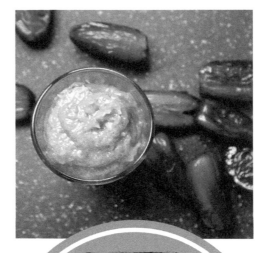

Putting it together

★ Blend all the ingredients in a food processor for about four or five minutes (until smooth). That's it.

Tricks and tips

For a thicker sauce, add less milk or more dates — this way, it becomes nice and spreadable, almost like dulce de leche.

★

Place in the microwave for about thirty seconds to create a hot toffee-like sauce.

★

Drizzle over courgette brownies.

★

For a hint of vanilla, use vanilla-flavoured soy milk.

Chocolate fudge

Growing up, we loved fudge, as most kids do. Finding a way to recreate its smooth, creamy texture without loads of sugar was a fun challenge.

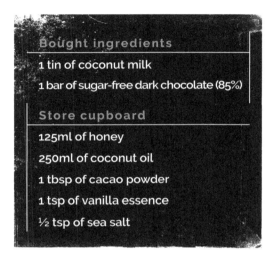

Bought ingredients

1 tin of coconut milk

1 bar of sugar-free dark chocolate (85%)

Store cupboard

125ml of honey

250ml of coconut oil

1 tbsp of cacao powder

1 tsp of vanilla essence

½ tsp of sea salt

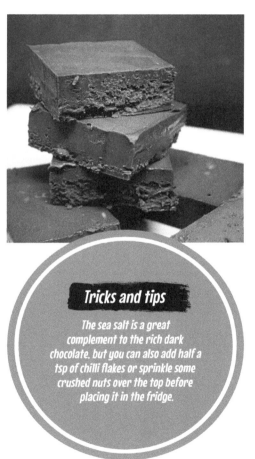

Putting it together

★ Break up the chocolate with your hands and place all the ingredients except the vanilla in a large saucepan on low heat.

★ Mix with a large wooden spoon until the chocolate has dissolved fully and everything is silky smooth. Let cool to room temperature and then stir in the vanilla essence.

★ Once the mixture has cooled, pour into a lined 20cm square baking tray and store in the fridge until set.

Tricks and tips

The sea salt is a great complement to the rich dark chocolate, but you can also add half a tsp of chilli flakes or sprinkle some crushed nuts over the top before placing it in the fridge.

Chocolate fudge cake

If you're looking to impress your friends, this is definitely the dessert for you. It's simple to make, and a showstopper.

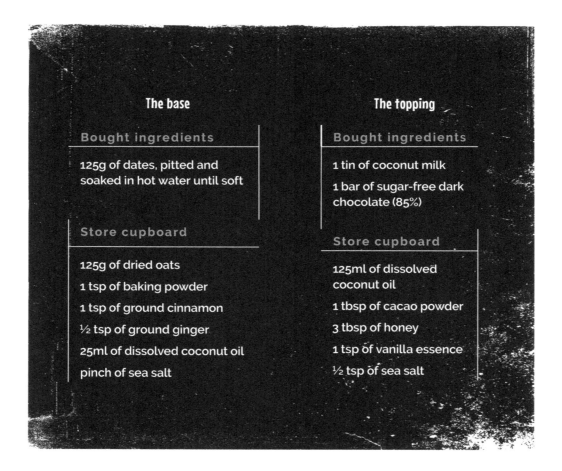

The base

Bought ingredients

125g of dates, pitted and soaked in hot water until soft

Store cupboard

125g of dried oats

1 tsp of baking powder

1 tsp of ground cinnamon

½ tsp of ground ginger

25ml of dissolved coconut oil

pinch of sea salt

The topping

Bought ingredients

1 tin of coconut milk

1 bar of sugar-free dark chocolate (85%)

Store cupboard

125ml of dissolved coconut oil

1 tbsp of cacao powder

3 tbsp of honey

1 tsp of vanilla essence

½ tsp of sea salt

To make the base

★ Preheat oven to 170 degrees Celsius and lightly oil a 20cm round cake tin.

★ Blend all the ingredients in a food processor until the dates are finely chopped — the coarseness of the base is up to you; we generally blend it until the pieces are quite small (for about thirty seconds to a minute, depending on the strength of your blender).

★ Press the mixture firmly into the bottom of the cake tin so that it forms an even crust.

★ Bake for fifteen to twenty minutes (until golden brown and biscuit-like).

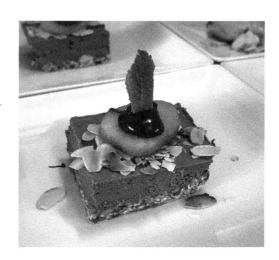

To make the topping

★ Place all the ingredients in a small saucepan and heat until the chocolate is melted. Stir continuously to make it nice and silky.

★ Once the chocolate has melted and the mixture is shiny, pour it over the base and place in the fridge for at least three or four hours. When it's set, the cake will have a soft, fudge-like texture.

★ Keep chilled until serving.

Tricks and tips

To evenly blitz the base, use the pulse button on your blender. This will help you control it more. You can also blend the mixture in batches if you find this easier (the only way to learn your easiest way is to try things out!).

★

We like to make this dessert the night before we serve it — this way, we know it will be properly set and will have the most amazing texture and consistency. This also makes it easier to slice.

★

You can place the cake in the freezer for a few hours, rather than in the fridge overnight, as this will help it to set faster.

Chocolate hummus

Yup, that's right — hummus! Chocolate hummus is ideal for chocolate-fondue night with a healthy twist.

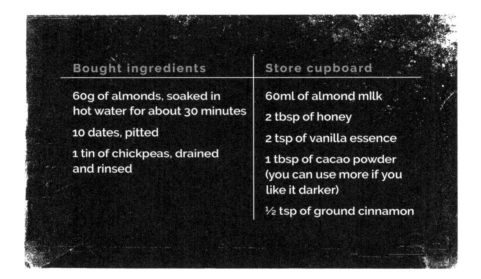

Bought ingredients	Store cupboard
60g of almonds, soaked in hot water for about 30 minutes	60ml of almond milk
10 dates, pitted	2 tbsp of honey
1 tin of chickpeas, drained and rinsed	2 tsp of vanilla essence
	1 tbsp of cacao powder (you can use more if you like it darker)
	½ tsp of ground cinnamon

Putting it together

★ Blend the almonds in a food processor with two of the dates and a splash of almond milk until the mixture has a thick, nut-butter consistency (this will take about five minutes).

★ Add the remaining ingredients and process until smooth.

★ Serve immediately with slices of fruit.

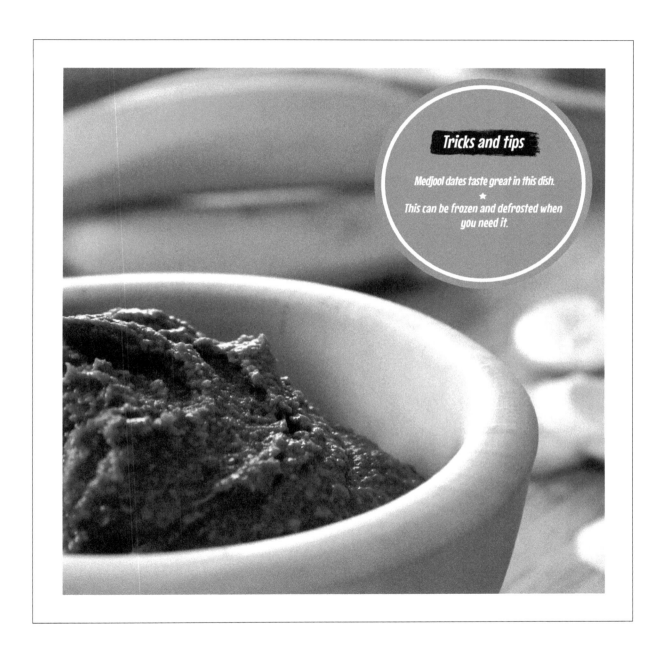

Tricks and tips

Medjool dates taste great in this dish.
★
This can be frozen and defrosted when you need it.

Coconut delight

Everyone loves a 'naughty' treat, and you don't have to feel guilty about eating this one.

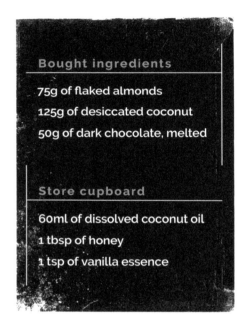

Bought ingredients

75g of flaked almonds

125g of desiccated coconut

50g of dark chocolate, melted

Store cupboard

60ml of dissolved coconut oil

1 tbsp of honey

1 tsp of vanilla essence

Putting it together

★ In a large mixing bowl, crush the almond flakes into small pieces (use your hands — this is the easiest way).

★ Add the desiccated coconut.

★ Melt the coconut oil in a small saucepan and add to the almonds and coconut in the bowl, along with the honey and vanilla essence.

★ Mix until everything is coated with the coconut oil.

★ Line a 15cm square baking tray with greaseproof paper and pour in the mixture. Press down so that it's about 2cm thick, and then place in the freezer for about thirty minutes (until it hardens).

★ Cut into squares then drizzle over the melted chocolate.

★ Place the bars on a plate lined with greaseproof paper and either return to the freezer or place them in the fridge until the chocolate hardens.

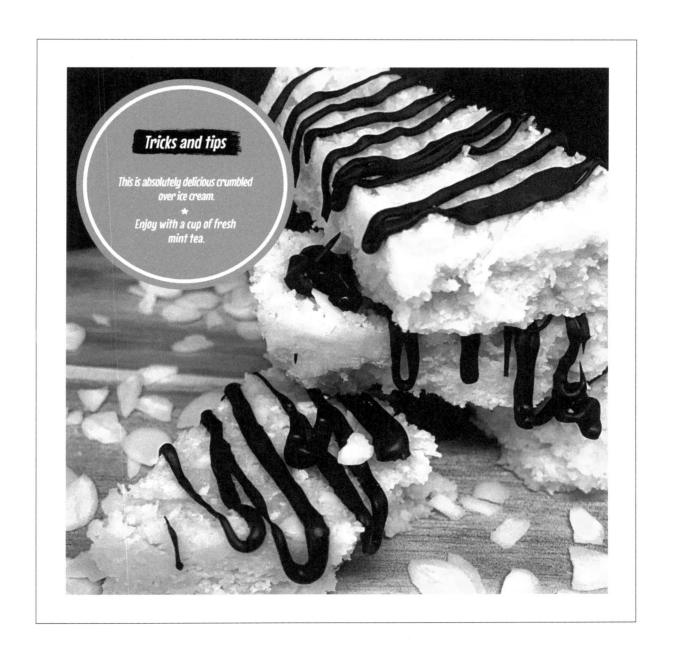

Tricks and tips

This is absolutely delicious crumbled over ice cream.

★

Enjoy with a cup of fresh mint tea.

Courgette and almond brownies

Bought ingredients	Store cupboard
300g of grated courgette	250g of chickpea flour
100g of almond flakes and 1 small handful for later use	1 tbsp of baking powder
20 dates, pitted	1 tbsp of cacao powder
125ml of almond or soy milk	1 tsp of ground ginger
2 eggs	2 tsp of vanilla essence
	60ml of dissolved coconut oil
	drizzle of honey

Putting it together

★ Preheat oven to 180 degrees Celsius and prepare a 25cm x 25cm baking tin — we line ours with greaseproof paper.

★ Remove as much excess fluid as possible from the grated courgette (place it in the middle of a clean dish towel and squeeze).

★ In a mixing bowl, combine the almond flakes, flour, baking powder, cacao powder, and ground ginger and mix until well blended.

★ Pour in the vanilla essence, coconut oil, and courgette and stir well.

★ In a food processer, .blend the dates and almond or soy milk until the mixture is caramel-like (this should take about three or four minutes). Pour into the cake mixture and mix well.

★ Separate the egg whites and whisk until stiff. Fold in the egg yolks, add to the cake mixture, and fold through.

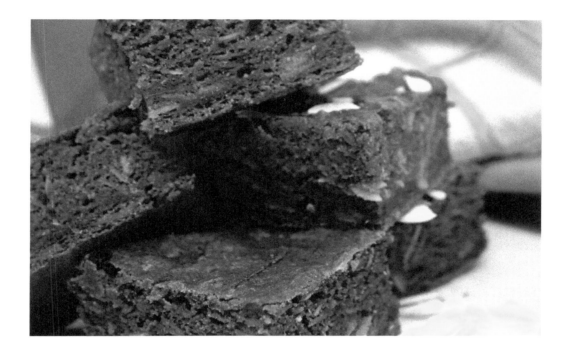

★ Pour the cake mixture into the baking tin, drizzle over a small amount of honey, and sprinkle over the handful of almond flakes.

★ Bake for twenty-five to thirty minutes (until the cake springs back when lightly touched or when a toothpick comes out clean).

★ Turn off the heat and let the cake stand in the oven for a further ten to fifteen minutes.

★ Remove, let cool, cut into squares, and serve.

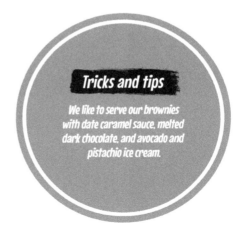

Tricks and tips

We like to serve our brownies with date caramel sauce, melted dark chocolate, and avocado and pistachio ice cream.

Courgette and apple muffins

These muffins are a tasty, quick, and easy snack for a pick-me-up.

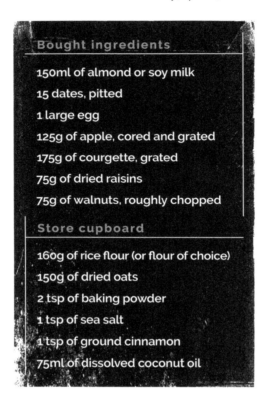

Bought ingredients

150ml of almond or soy milk

15 dates, pitted

1 large egg

125g of apple, cored and grated

175g of courgette, grated

75g of dried raisins

75g of walnuts, roughly chopped

Store cupboard

160g of rice flour (or flour of choice)

150g of dried oats

2 tsp of baking powder

1 tsp of sea salt

1 tsp of ground cinnamon

75ml of dissolved coconut oil

Putting it together

★ Preheat oven to 200 degrees Celsius and prepare a standard 12-cup muffin tray by either spraying with cooking spray or lining with paper cups.

★ In a large bowl, combine the flour, oats, baking powder, salt, and cinnamon and mix until everything is well blended.

★ Blend the milk, dates, and coconut oil in a blender until smooth and creamy.

★ In a separate bowl, beat the egg. (We sometimes separate the white from the yolk and whisk separately because this makes it a lot fluffier than if you whisk the egg whole, which then gives you a nice, light-textured muffin.)

★ Add the egg and date-milk to the flour mixture and mix well.

★ Add the apple, courgette, raisins, and walnuts and mix gently and thoroughly with a wooden spoon. The batter will be thick and lumpy.

★ Spoon the mixture into the muffin cups and bake for about twenty-five minutes, or until the muffins begin to brown and a toothpick poked into the centre of them comes out clean.

★ Remove the muffins from the pan and let cool on a wire rack.

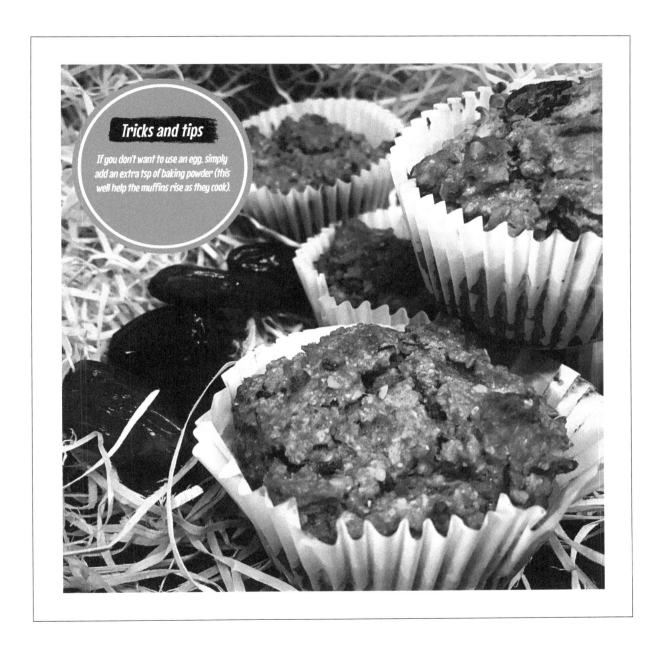

Tricks and tips

If you don't want to use an egg, simply add an extra tsp of baking powder (this well help the muffins rise as they cook).

Cranberry granola bar

A retreat favourite that's packed full of nutrients and flavour.

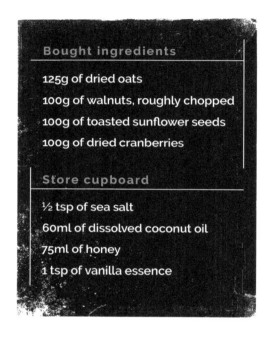

Bought ingredients

125g of dried oats

100g of walnuts, roughly chopped

100g of toasted sunflower seeds

100g of dried cranberries

Store cupboard

½ tsp of sea salt

60ml of dissolved coconut oil

75ml of honey

1 tsp of vanilla essence

Putting it together

★ Preheat oven to 180 degrees Celsius and line a square baking tray with greaseproof paper.

★ Lightly toast the oats and walnuts (you can also add the sunflower seeds if they aren't toasted) in a large heated frying pan with the sea salt for a few minutes, gently tossing every now and then so that they don't catch.

★ While your oats and nuts are toasting, place the coconut oil, honey, and vanilla essence in a small bowl and heat in the microwave for about thirty seconds. This will make the mixing much easier.

★ In a large bowl, mix the toasted oats and nuts, sunflower seeds, cranberries, and honey mixture in a large bowl until everything is nicely coated and sticky.

★ Pour the mixture into the baking tray and press firmly so that it's packed nice and tight.

★ Bake for about ten minutes (until it starts to turn golden brown).

★ Remove from the oven and, using a spatula or the back of a large wooden spoon, press down the mixture to pack it more firmly.

★ Let cool down, remove from baking tray, and cut into squares.

★ Store in an airtight container at room temperature.

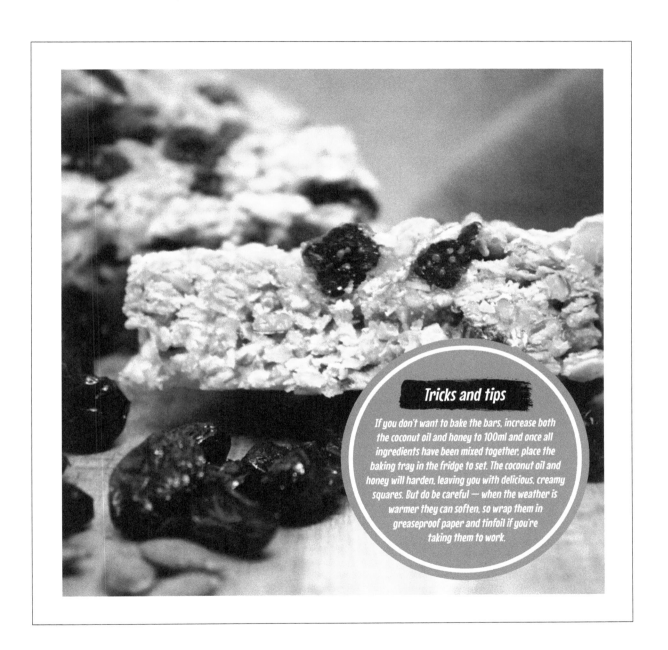

Tricks and tips

If you don't want to bake the bars, increase both the coconut oil and honey to 100ml and once all ingredients have been mixed together, place the baking tray in the fridge to set. The coconut oil and honey will harden, leaving you with delicious, creamy squares. But do be careful — when the weather is warmer they can soften, so wrap them in greaseproof paper and tinfoil if you're taking them to work.

D-Toxd fruit salad and yogurt

After every juice cleanse at the retreat, the first 'meal' that people have is this delicious treat. It's so simple to prepare and is one of the highlights of the week.

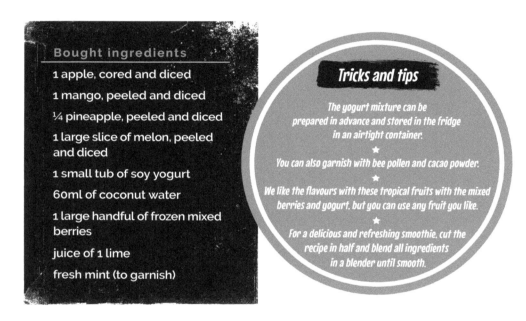

Bought ingredients

1 apple, cored and diced

1 mango, peeled and diced

¼ pineapple, peeled and diced

1 large slice of melon, peeled and diced

1 small tub of soy yogurt

60ml of coconut water

1 large handful of frozen mixed berries

juice of 1 lime

fresh mint (to garnish)

Tricks and tips

The yogurt mixture can be prepared in advance and stored in the fridge in an airtight container.

★

You can also garnish with bee pollen and cacao powder.

★

We like the flavours with these tropical fruits with the mixed berries and yogurt, but you can use any fruit you like.

★

For a delicious and refreshing smoothie, cut the recipe in half and blend all ingredients in a blender until smooth.

Putting it together

★ In a large bowl, combine the diced fruit and mix well.

★ Blend the yogurt, coconut water, mixed berries, and lime juice in a blender for twenty to thirty seconds (until creamy).

★ Pour blended yogurt mixture into a bowl and gently spoon over some of the mixed fruit salad.

★ Garnish with fresh mint and enjoy.

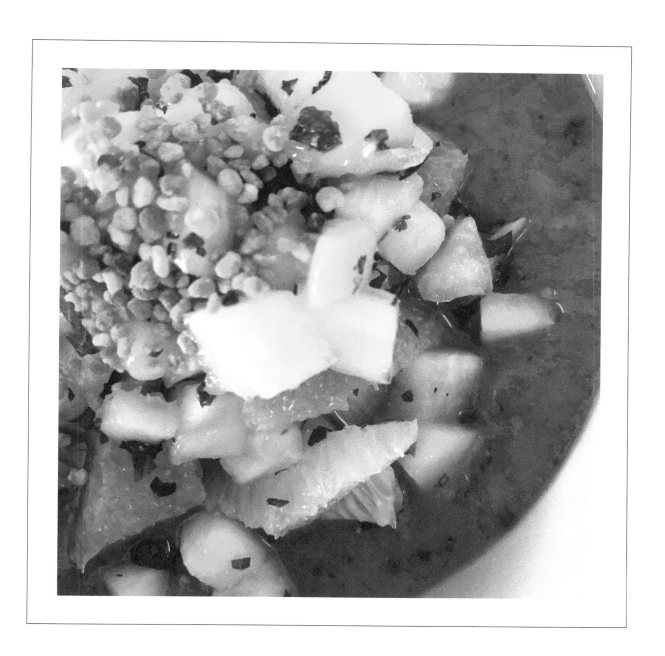

D-Toxd hummus

We don't really like tahini, the nutty ingredient that gives hummus its traditional flavour, so we decided to create our own recipe for the spread.

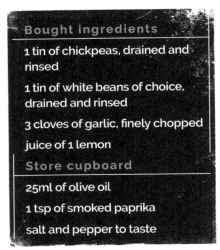

Bought ingredients

1 tin of chickpeas, drained and rinsed

1 tin of white beans of choice, drained and rinsed

3 cloves of garlic, finely chopped

juice of 1 lemon

Store cupboard

25ml of olive oil

1 tsp of smoked paprika

salt and pepper to taste

Putting it together

★ In a blender, blitz all ingredients to desired consistency. If you feel your hummus is too thick, add a little oil or water.

We also like to play around with the recipe and try out these variations:

Spicy

★ Add a small chilli (or two) while blending your ingredients.

★ Use hot paprika instead of the smoked version.

Roasted red pepper

★ Making lasagna for dinner? The hummus is a perfect accompaniment. Roast an extra red pepper and add it to the blender for a touch of sweetness. The red pepper goes well with the smoked paprika.

Pesto

★ Substitute the smoked paprika for two large tbsp of green pesto. The cheesy taste complements the chickpeas. This version is quite refreshing!

★ If you don't want to use shop-bought pesto, add a handful of fresh basil, some grated Parmesan cheese, and a few pine nuts while blending.

Green

★ Add a small tin of garden peas to the blend. A small amount of mint and a little extra lemon juice will give it a fresh taste — and will make it look great, too.

Beetroot

★ Beetroot is a great source of nutrients, and it's perfect for cleansing the blood and giving you a boost. Roast some beetroot and add to the blend.

★ You can do the same with carrots — drizzle with a small amount of honey and a squeeze of lemon juice before roasting. These are slightly sweeter variations.

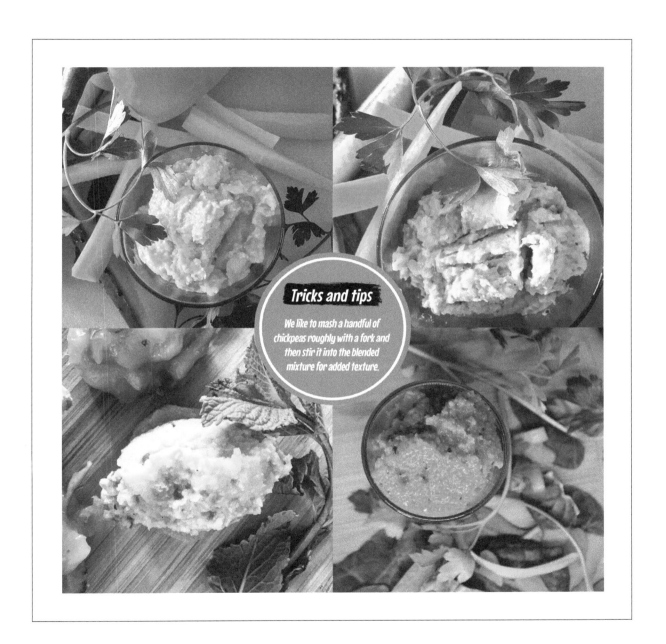

Tricks and tips

We like to mash a handful of chickpeas roughly with a fork and then stir it into the blended mixture for added texture.

D-Toxd mixed nuts and fruit

These days, you can easily buy packs of nuts and fruit. But sometimes, it's fun to make your own. And this way, you know exactly what you're getting.

Bought ingredients	Store cupboard
100g of walnuts	1 tsp of solid coconut oil
100g of almonds	1 tbsp of honey
100g of pumpkin seeds	1 tsp of sea salt
100g of sunflower seeds	½ tsp of dried chilli flakes
100g of goji berries	1 tsp of cacao powder

Putting it together

★ Chop the walnuts and almonds. In a large frying pan, lightly heat the coconut oil and honey. Toss in the nuts and pumpkin and sunflower seeds and lightly toast (mix them around until they begin to slightly change colour). Let cool.

★ While the nuts are toasting, mix the sea salt (we like to crush it between our fingers so that the flakes break down into small pieces), chilli flakes, and cacao powder in a small bowl.

★ Pour the cooled nuts and seeds into a mixing bowl, sprinkle over the goji berries and mixed spices, and toss until everything is evenly coated.

★ Store in an airtight container.

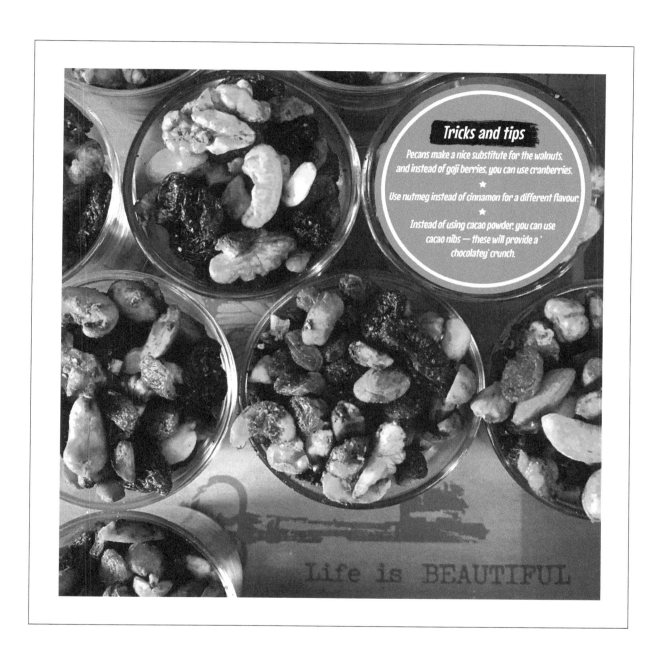

Tricks and tips

Pecans make a nice substitute for the walnuts, and instead of goji berries, you can use cranberries.

★

Use nutmeg instead of cinnamon for a different flavour.

★

Instead of using cacao powder, you can use cacao nibs — these will provide a ' chocolatey' crunch.

Life is BEAUTIFUL

D-Toxd Peanut Butter bars

This treat is really, really, *really* yum! And what makes us love it even more is that it's full of nutrition.

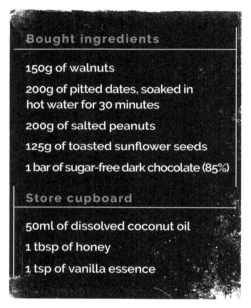

Bought ingredients

150g of walnuts

200g of pitted dates, soaked in hot water for 30 minutes

200g of salted peanuts

125g of toasted sunflower seeds

1 bar of sugar-free dark chocolate (85%)

Store cupboard

50ml of dissolved coconut oil

1 tbsp of honey

1 tsp of vanilla essence

Putting it together

★ Line a 20cm x 20cm baking tray with greaseproof paper.

★ Blend the walnuts and dates in a food processor until the mixture is dough-like.

★ Tightly pack the 'dough' in the baking tray. Place in the freezer while you prepare the peanut butter.

★ Blend the peanuts, coconut oil, vanilla essence and honey in the food processor for about a minute and then scrape down the sides. We used pre-toasted salted peanuts to save time.

★ Blend again for another two to three minutes (until the nuts break down and form a smooth mixture). It might appear as if nothing is happening, but after a while, a butter texture is created. If the mixture is too dry, add a little extra coconut oil.

★ In a bowl, mix the peanut butter with the toasted sunflower seeds.

★ Remove the baking tray from the freezer, spread over the peanut butter mixture, and return to the freezer for ten to fifteen minutes.

★ Melt the chocolate in a heatproof bowl set over a pan of simmering water and then pour the chocolate over the peanut butter mixture.

★ Return to the freezer for about thirty minutes to set firmly.

★ Remove from baking tray and cut into squares.

★ Store in the freezer or fridge if you're not going to serve it straight away, or else it will start to melt.

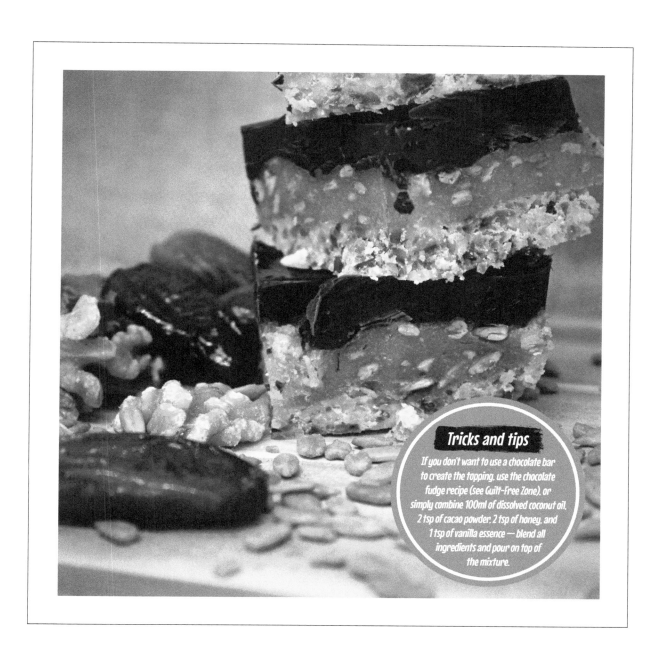

Tricks and tips

If you don't want to use a chocolate bar to create the topping, use the chocolate fudge recipe (see Guilt-Free Zone), or simply combine 100ml of dissolved coconut oil, 2 tsp of cacao powder, 2 tsp of honey, and 1 tsp of vanilla essence — blend all ingredients and pour on top of the mixture.

Energy balls

These are great when you're on the run and need a quick boost of energy.

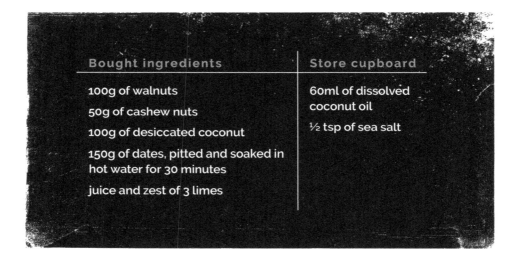

Bought ingredients	Store cupboard
100g of walnuts	60ml of dissolved coconut oil
50g of cashew nuts	½ tsp of sea salt
100g of desiccated coconut	
150g of dates, pitted and soaked in hot water for 30 minutes	
juice and zest of 3 limes	

Putting it together

★ Place the walnuts and cashew nuts in a food processor and pulse until finely chopped — you don't want to process them too much or make them too fine.

★ Add the remaining ingredients except for half of the desiccated coconut and repeat the process until the mixture starts to come together into a large ball.

★ Form ball shapes by rolling 1 tbsp of the mixture between your palms.

★ Gently roll each ball in the remaining coconut until it's lightly coated and store in an airtight container in the fridge for up to a week.

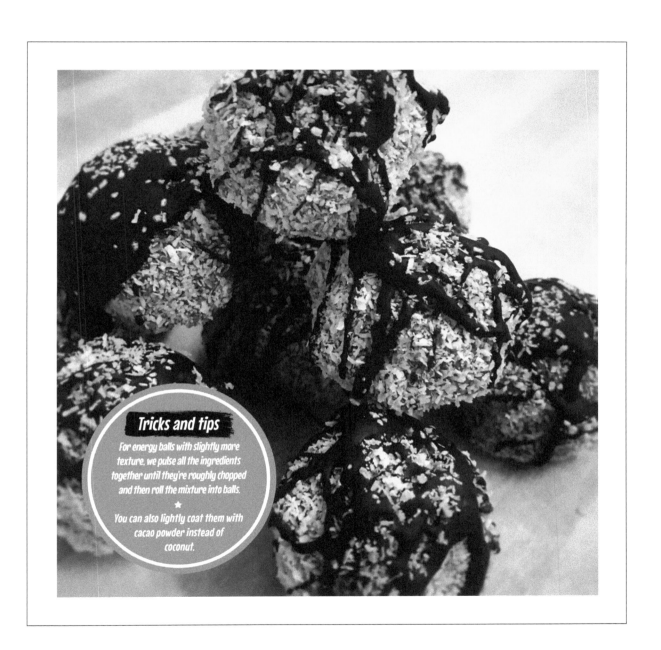

Tricks and tips

For energy balls with slightly more texture, we pulse all the ingredients together until they're roughly chopped and then roll the mixture into balls.

★

You can also lightly coat them with cacao powder instead of coconut.

Quick and easy guacamole

A healthy option for a quick and easy snack.

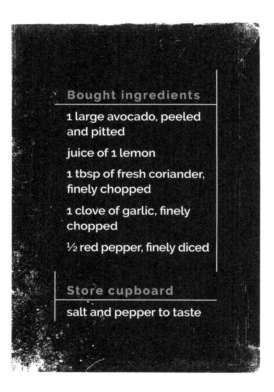

Bought ingredients

1 large avocado, peeled and pitted

juice of 1 lemon

1 tbsp of fresh coriander, finely chopped

1 clove of garlic, finely chopped

½ red pepper, finely diced

Store cupboard

salt and pepper to taste

Putting it together

★ Place the avocado in a bowl with the lemon juice, coriander, and garlic and blend with a handheld blender. If you don't have one, simply mash it with a fork.

★ Once desired consistency is achieved, simply stir through the red pepper with a fork.

★ Season to taste.

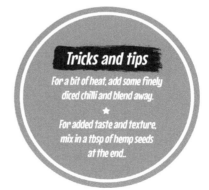

Tricks and tips

For a bit of heat, add some finely diced chilli and blend away.

★

For added taste and texture, mix in a tbsp of hemp seeds at the end..

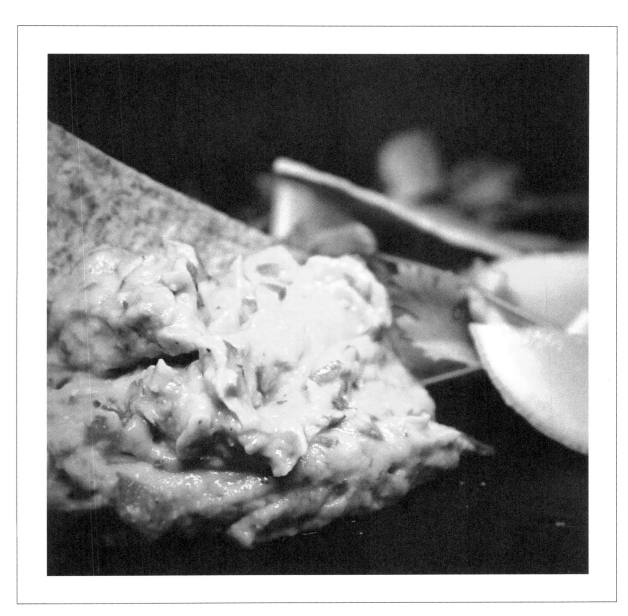

The FUEL Challenge

It's not what you say you're going to do that matters. It's what you do right now that truly counts.

What you have in your hands is over two years of tireless and continual hard work. There were times when, quite simply, we didn't want to carry on; times when we simply thought, 'What on earth is the point of doing all of this?'

We hadn't realised how much was involved in putting something like this together, and had we known at the start, we more than likely wouldn't have opened our mouths. But we truly believe in FUEL and The Bouncing Chef. We live our lives by the FUEL philosophy, and we want to share it with the world. After all, what's the point of learning something, getting results in your life, and not sharing the knowledge? That's just plain selfish.

So here's the question we really want to ask you:

Are you going to be one of those people who puts the book down and carries on doing the same things while hoping for a different result?

Or are you going to put the principles into action?

If you're in the latter group of people, what we've put together on our website will help you do just this. When we started our first coaching business, in 2010, we created a ten-day challenge to help people create new habits. Today, we still use the document we created for this challenge.

We had those doubts in the backs of our heads — 'This is too simple to be effective' — but for once, we chose not to listen. After a few days, we began to hear back from people taking part in the challenge. They shared personal insights and revelations, and since then, we've continued to use the challenge's simple principles in all the work we do with clients. We've seen people turn their lives inside out as a result.

Recently, we've refreshed and updated everything. Up for the challenge?

See you soon, then.

To take part, visit www.thebouncingchef.com/thefuelchallenge

Acknowledgements

We would like to say a very big thank you to the people who have helped us to make this crazy dream a reality. Your support and encouragement have inspired us to keep on keeping on. This book is dedicated to you all.

Thank you from the bottom of our bouncing hearts.

The Big Man — our CEO and the one in charge of everything: you give us strength and courage to share a simple message of fun and friendship.

Mirjam (Jeroen's wife) and Kerry-Leigh (Gareth's sister): without you two wonderful ladies constantly pushing us forward, who knows where we would be?

Darryn, Savannah, Luca, and Lola: you are the world's most wonderful children and the driving force behind everything we do.

Julia W: you've been our helping, guiding, supporting hand in creating the magic of the Bouncing Chef.

Jane Milton and her amazing team: thank you for testing everything for us to make sure it's as good as it can be, and for believing in this right from the start.

Anne S and "Bean": thank you for sharing some of your delicious meals with us and inspiring us to include them for people to enjoy too.

Dan M, Shaa W and Paul B: thank you for being our virtual coaches, keeping us on track, focused, and pressing on even when we felt like throwing the towel in.

The following people also contributed to making this all happen: Linda Keller, Keith MacLennan, Liz Gibney, Michele Leathley, Helen Brough, John and Ann Hardy, Gemma Skillett, Theresa Thompson, Tessa Messaoudi, Kingsley Duffy, Bev Pinnell, Sanchia Franks, Liz Lavin, Kathy West, Noeleen M, Marie Flanagan, Nicole Prins, Reilly Phillips, Lulu Bott, Tony and Priya Miles, Tracy Smith, Sue Verstage, Mikey and Mariann Johnson, Denise Duignan, Julia Webster, Sarah Duce, Denise Fleming, Alison Talbot, Jane Donachy, Jane Pascoe, Mike and Emily Edge, Veerle Leemen, Sue Gibbons, and Alison Hunter.

The Authors

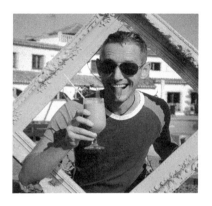 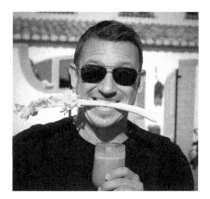

Imagine waking up from a coma and being told by the doctor that you should be dead. In 2002, this was Gareth's reality. He was hooked up to a life-support machine and restrained to a hospital bed. This was the turning point for him.

After a life of drug addiction, eating disorders, and mental health problems, he finally realised at the age of twenty-nine that he'd been given a second chance — a chance to make massive changes. It was now or never. He decided to leave his home in Zimbabwe and travel to London, to learn more about himself and to study.

Jeroen had a different problem. To overcome his problems with drugs and an unhealthy lifestyle following a turbulent childhood, he was damaging himself through excessive exercise — something that is very common in today's world.

Jeroen was travelling between London and Holland for work, and finally realised that living out of a suitcase wasn't doing anything for his mental health or his addiction to exercise.

He too began to educate himself in a different way, and it was at a course in London in 2009 that Jeroen met Gareth.

Their common desire to help other people brought them together not only as friends, but also as founders of a health retreat in Spain, D-Toxd, which is now in its fifth year.

The Bouncing Chef is who they are together and represents everything they are truly passionate about: fitness, food and, most of all, fun.

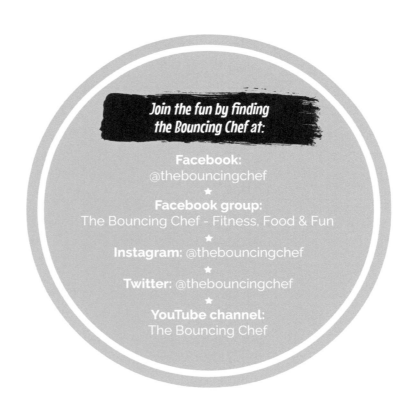

Join the fun by finding the Bouncing Chef at:

Facebook:
@thebouncingchef

★

Facebook group:
The Bouncing Chef - Fitness, Food & Fun

★

Instagram: @thebouncingchef

★

Twitter: @thebouncingchef

★

YouTube channel:
The Bouncing Chef

Lightning Source UK Ltd.
Milton Keynes UK
UKHW05f0916080718
325385UK00005B/17/P